Birth, Boobs and

Birth, Boobs and Bad Advice

Published by Two Hoots 2012
© Zoe Kleinman

email breastfeedingbattles@gmail.com
www.birthboobsandbadadvice.wordpress.com
ISBN 978-0-9574756-0-1

*For women everywhere who find themselves here.
And for Reece and Harrison, who never gave up on me.*

Birth, Boobs and Bad Advice

'*All animals are equal, but some are more equal than others.*'

GEORGE ORWELL, ANIMAL FARM

IN THE BEGINNING...

The last text I sent pre-birth was to my sister Aimee.

It's starting to really fucking hurt now, I wrote, and I must have meant it because the text is signed off with lots of little c's instead of x's by mistake. Ordinarily these virtual kisses between my sibling and I are notable only in their absence, which generally means that the sender is royally pissed off with the recipient.

Oh God!! she replied. *Drugs??*

I was on my way to the hospital with a big, firm belly, broken waters and, according to the clock on the car stereo, contractions that were three minutes apart. I was secretly looking forward to checking in and chowing down on some serious meds. I had already decided to try them all and I was increasingly certain about that. Not for me a natural birth.

'Bring on the pharmaceuticals,' I had silently cheered during the pain-relief lesson in our antenatal classes (sandwiched as it was between knitted boobs and the bizarre revelation that the size to which the cervix must open during childbirth is EXACTLY the same as that of a box of cheese triangles. This fact still haunts me, particularly when in the dairy aisle during the weekly shop).

I gripped the handrail and prayed for a tractor-free journey as my husband, Reece, and I raced down country roads to the county hospital. By the time we got there it was 9.30 p.m.

A friendly midwife sat with me as I explained how I felt and that I'd woken up that morning with what felt like period pain which had got progressively stronger. I'd cleaned the house, popped into town for lunch and even had laminate flooring laid in the lounge (I stopped short of laying it myself – I am very much a creature of comfort when it comes to DIY at the best of times, and being 40 weeks pregnant hadn't changed that). At that point, a post-nap trip to the bathroom revealed that things were progressing more rapidly than I had thought.

Not rapidly enough, though, according to the duty midwife.

'You'll be having this baby in the next forty-eight hours,' she told me as I instinctively bounced on a gym ball in an empty delivery room and felt, on what would become the first of many occasions, that nagging feeling that my instinct was at odds with the professional view. On a scale of one to a hundred, my pain level was about a seven, she said. She seemed to know this simply by checking my blood pressure, which was impressively intuitive. Perhaps she was also good at Tarot, although I didn't think to ask at the time.

'Would you like to see a picture of a woman who's REALLY in labour?' she asked, possibly sensing my disbelief. Because by this time things were really, really, really fucking hurting.

'Yup, that's exactly what I need right now,' I muttered through clenched, well, everything.

Her suggestion that I go back home (a 45-minute drive away), have a bath (I hate our bath), go to bed (I can't sleep in a room with a ticking clock in it, let alone with 20 contractions an hour) and come back in the morning was not well received. Eventually we agreed that as it was quiet in the maternity unit that night, I could stay there. I was pathetically grateful. We decided to fill the birthing pool for me to relax in before popping a sleeping pill and passing out. Every synapse in my body was screaming that this was not the way this night was going to pan out, but I decided to play along.

The midwife went off to fill the pool and I shut myself in the bathroom. I liked the enclosed space and I really liked sitting on the loo which, with hindsight, must have been the whole 'bearing down' thing that women talk about in mum-to-be online chat rooms (I have lurked on several hundred. Did you know they actually have their own language? FTM – first time mum, DH – darling husband, MIL/SIL – mother-/sister-in-law etc. Also they go on about 'sticky baby dust' a lot, which I think is supposed to mean good luck with the pregnancy but sounds pretty gross when you think about it).

Anyway. By now the pain was making me retch and the little gas and air I tried to have just made me feel even sicker. My husband had the sense to look sympathetic when I told him it wasn't working.

I'm going to die when I get into the teens on this painometer, let alone a hundred, I thought miserably. *I'll die in childbirth like a Victorian scullery maid and the baby will be brought up by Reece and his second wife, who'll be thinner yet more buxom than me, with better hair, and my child will never know she's not really his mother.*

Actually I didn't think any of that. I just thought, OUCH! But under ordinary circumstances that is precisely the kind of dark shit I can come up with to give myself a hard time over.

Finally I got in the pool and for about half an hour it did make me feel a bit better. The lights were dimmed and Michael Parkinson was playing easy-listening classics on Radio 2 (odd that he will now be forever synonymous with childbirth in my mind. A couple of weeks later a camera zoomed in on him in the crowd during the men's final at Wimbledon and I swear my uterus involuntarily spasmed). Reece was tactfully ignoring the fact that blood clots were slowly joining me in my languid flotation tank.

Suddenly the contractions became more... pushy.

'I need the loo again,' I gasped and ran as fast as a labouring woman can run into the en suite bathroom. Because the blood clots were one thing but there was NO WAY my 'DH' was going to watch me splashing about in a pool of my own poo.

I decided that the pool and I had had our fun and the midwife helped me hobble back to the delivery room. At this point, two and a half hours after I arrived, she decided to do an internal examination.

'Oh my God,' she said. 'You're eight centimetres dilated. I can feel the head!'

'Oh,' I said, brightening and remembering the Dairylea. 'Does that mean it's time for my epidural?'

'This baby is coming NOW,' said the midwife firmly in reply. This apparently signified my having completely missed the window of opportunity for any drugs whatsoever.

According to Reece, I spent the remaining 90 minutes of my labour muttering 'I told you it hurt' in between some seriously primal howling that I didn't even realise I was capable of. The midwife later apologised to me, by the way, and told me that I must be a 'silent labourer', which made me feel very Victorian once again.

At one point she told me to make a 'moo' noise like a cow – something I vaguely remembered from a hippy birth book my friend had given me (apparently the sound relaxes your throat, which in turn relaxes other, erm, passages). Despite this, I didn't really fancy re-enacting Old McDonald's farm in the latter stages of active labour. After much coaxing I relented – grudgingly.

'Fucking moooooo!' I screamed during one particularly agonising contraction. It actually did make me smile – no mean feat when you feel like an extra from *Prometheus* (the sci-fi film, not the guy who had his liver picked out by the birds. Close call, though).

The only pain relief I was given – and I was genuinely grateful for it, even though in the cold light of day it is pretty weird – was frankincense oil. Seriously. There I was in a modern hospital in 21st-century Britain giving birth with the aid of something straight out of the Old Testament. Still, if it was good enough for Jesus... (I don't recall any gold being on offer, though. Just as well they didn't break out the myrrh. I have no idea what that actually is.)

Baby Harrison was born at 1.29 a.m. on 21 June. For an utterly agonising second or two, which felt like a lifetime, there was silence. And then he opened his little mouth and uttered his first cry. From that moment I was utterly, uncontrollably overwhelmed with love for this tiny man, and I knew my life would never be the same again because I would never want to be far from him. From now on nothing would ever be more important to me than this small bundle with his huge, shiny eyes.

'Hello, darling,' I whispered between happy tears. 'I am so glad you're here.'

My arms ached to hold him and the chemical memory of every single painful contraction began to ebb calmly away. I never believed those women who say you forget the agony of labour, but for me it turned out to be true. These days I do remember that it hurt like hell, frankly, but not specifically how.

Unfortunately within minutes we witnessed the sort of behaviour that led me to write all of this down in the first place.

Firstly Reece suddenly realised that they were about to cut the umbilical cord without saying a word, and he had expressly said he wished to do it himself. Then – without even asking me – I was given an injection of Syntometrine to make me deliver the placenta straight away. It is supposed to be a choice thing. Again, not a word was said, but I know I felt that jab in my thigh and two seconds later the placenta arrived.

A paediatrician turned up (I forget why) and she placed the baby on a glorified hot plate to warm him up. The midwife bristled and an argument openly erupted between them about whether the baby should be warming himself on my chest instead. Then the doctor who arrived to do my stitches (giving birth really is a gruesome business) incurred the midwife's wrath further by asking her to clean my traumatised lower half afterwards.

'Don't bother finishing the job yourself then,' she spat as he beat a hasty retreat.

Reece and I exchanged glances. I felt incredibly euphoric, wired beyond belief on endorphins and hormones and no bloody artificial stimulants whatsoever (can you tell that I am still a tad bitter about that?), and this strange little display of office politics felt wildly incongruous with my otherworldly state. In short, it was in danger of seriously messing with my mellow.

So you see for me, the postnatal care I received was decidedly rocky from the get-go. When I was pregnant I focused all my energy on worrying about the birth. Specifically the pain and the endless potential complications. It never occurred to me that the really scary shit would happen afterwards.

But as time went on, I started to think that despite the fact that I was a hugely emotional and overtired FTM (on the day I wrote this introduction I had quite literally cried over spilt milk: Reece came home to find me in a pool of tears over a puddle of semi-skimmed), somebody needed to look into the way in which we provide postnatal care, because it seemed to me that something was seriously amiss.

And all that was before we knew I was going to have enormous problems with breastfeeding.

CHAPTER 1

A Brief History Lesson

Friends who had already had children had warned us about the 'breastapo' – the 'breast is best' evangelists for whom there simply is no other way of feeding an infant. They lurk everywhere, in hospitals, cafes and shops, with metaphorically wagging fingers and undisguised contempt for those mums either unable or unwilling to get their baps out on demand.

If you're feeling particularly masochistic, try using the loyalty card schemes of either Boots or Sainsbury's to buy formula milk. I think I'd have received a warmer reception if I'd walked up to the till and put bomb-making equipment on the counter. It is 'against company policy', I was told, to include baby formula products in the loyalty scheme at Boots because it goes against the promotion of breastfeeding. Interestingly no such moral high ground is evident when it comes to nutritionally dubious and horrendously overpriced weight-loss supplements, or the myriad of expensive elixirs of eternal youth (moisturisers to the likes of you and me) also on sale.

Boots says the no-formula rule is the result of an EU directive that penalises anybody offering an 'incentive' to not breastfeed. This is presumably the same EU that used to place size and shape restrictions on 36 varieties of fruits and vegetables, and in 2010 got the world's chicken owners into a flap with some draft legislation which seemed to suggest that selling eggs by the dozen should be banned (it wasn't). Yup, they are clearly watching our backs – cheers Brussels. Without you we'd all be strangely shaped, non-lactating zombies staggering around supermarkets and killing anyone who stood between us and our next fix of inappropriately labelled dairy products.

I certainly wasn't deprived of breastfeeding 'support'. It constituted around 80 per cent of my postnatal care. It just didn't work. Pretty much everything else came secondary to the three-hourly feeding schedule (much more on that anon). My tiny son and I dutifully worked our way through a veritable Karma Sutra of breastfeeding positions during my six-day hospital stay, the sole purpose of which was to 'establish breastfeeding'. If I'd had £1 for every midwife who said 'Have you tried holding him under your arm like a rugby ball?' I could have bought an entire scrum half by now.

According to the sweetly acronymed NICE – the National Institute for Health and Clinical Excellence – the core principles of current postnatal care guidelines, which include the unequivocal hammering home of the breast-is-best message, have been around for some time. A report by academics from Leicester University in 2006, available on the NICE website, states that:

> Current models of postnatal care originate from the beginning of the 20th century.... The timing and content of care have altered little since then despite a dramatic reduction in mortality rates which occurred around the middle of the 20th century.

Woah. The early 20th century? Okay, in that case let's take a little leap back through time.

Back in 1911, 110 babies out of every 1,000 in the UK died before they reached their first birthday. By 1951, this figure had fallen to 21 per 1,000, and by 2001, it was just 6 per 1,000.

In 1911, a curious tome called *The Woman's Book: Contains Everything a Woman Ought to Know* was published (you can still buy it, by the way, although these days it's the kind of thing you'd give a mate for a laugh at her hen do or baby shower rather than a serious guide to life – I hope). *The Female Eunuch* it ain't.

It includes a section on recommended 'nursery recipes' – mouth-watering delights such as 'barley water' – literally the strained water from boiled pearl barley; albumen water, a scrumptious concoction of egg white, water and sugar; and whey – half a pint of milk and half a pint of rennet. Sit me on a tuffet and fetch me a spider, already. Even culinary siren Nigella Lawson would struggle to make any of that sound appealing. No wonder breast was bloody best.

However, while the babies were busy with their barley banquets, their parents weren't exactly getting their five-a-day either. According to the British Library:

> At the beginning of the century the English population ate very poorly. In 1917, when 2,500,000 men from across the social spectrum were given medical examinations, over forty per cent of them were found to be unfit for military service – mainly due to malnourishment.

I actually had to read that several times – they are pretty staggering statistics. Especially when you consider that presumably the menfolk were being fed by their wives and mothers, which means that the women were more than likely similarly malnourished. So let's assume 40 per cent of husbands AND WIVES were malnourished.

People who are malnourished have this annoying tendency to be more prone to illness, so getting antibodies from your mother via breast milk was definitely a good survival tactic. Although how much breastmilk a malnourished mother could produce is questionable, and while formula has been around since 1867, it has never been cheap. No wonder infant – and maternal for that matter – mortality was so high.

(By the way, in 2009 the British Association for Parenteral and Enteral Nutrition released a report claiming that 3 million people in the whole of the UK – 1.9 per cent of a population of nearly 62 million – were either malnourished or 'at risk' from malnourishment.)

But from 100 years ago, when 40 per cent of the population was potentially eating depressingly badly, spring the basics of modern postnatal care. Food for thought, if you'll pardon the pun.

CHAPTER 2

A Book at Bedtime

Meanwhile, back at the hospital, I was already struggling. I had my own room, which was delightful – at least I only had one baby to keep me awake rather than the four mothers and babies who can share each postnatal ward room, I thought. The maternity unit was quiet while I was there, so I never left my L-shaped 'delivery suite', which for some reason was named 'Cranborne'. This made it sound a bit posh and penthousey and private healthcarish, which could not have been further from the truth.

An NHS curtain was tactfully drawn across the actual 'delivery' bit, but I still took disbelieving peeks at it (if those stirrups could talk...) and a couple of times my exhausted husband actually took an afternoon nap on the bed itself, which had obviously been cleaned up a lot since Harrison exploded into the world in a torrent of blood (mine) and poo (his, I hope).

Reece brought me a big stash of my favourite 'real-life stories' magazines to read. Professionally I'm a journalist for a serious news organisation, but privately I have long been a sucker for the sort of headlines I will never get to write – 'I Grew a Third Kneecap Under My Chin!' and 'Turkish Love Rats on Parade'. I used to take these mags to the doctors' surgery when I had finished with them until I noticed that they never seemed to make it into the waiting room. Perhaps because they also tend to contain a few utterly harrowing health dramas.

Those aside, I intended to fight off the baby blues with the ever-entertaining Readers' Top Tips pages that inevitably crop up in one form or another in these titles. I am always cheered by the upbeat helpful hints: 'Instead of wasting money on expensive wallpaper, why not make your own? All you need is a reporter's notebook and a felt-tip pen!', especially when the contributor has included a terrible picture of their own efforts.

At this time, though, I was too tired and emotional to even open the magazines, to be honest, but I was glad they were there because there wasn't a huge variety of alternative reading material in my room. There were two big posters about the benefits of breastfeeding on the toilet door and one very glossy, jovial leaflet in cartoon yellow, pink and blue called 'Off to the Best Start', which was all about, you guessed it, breastfeeding.

Here's a quick summary:

Page 1 – breastfeeding helps protect your baby from infection and strengthens the bond between you (formula does NOT).
Page 2 – if you do NOT breastfeed here are seven major illnesses your baby might get (a hypochondriac's dream, ranging from diarrhoea to diabetes).
Page 3 – benefits of breastfeeding for mother (this, shamelessly, even includes weight loss because all women are obsessed with their figures, right?).
Page 4 – after your baby is born... guess what?... start breastfeeding!
Pages 5, 6, 7 – how to breastfeed.
Pages 8, 9 – signs that your baby is feeding well, including an enormous picture of a happy infant with a mouthful of anonymous breast.
Pages 10, 11 – top tips; first one: 'Try not to give your baby other food or drink.'
Pages 12, 13, 14 – expressing breast milk.
Page 15 – how do I know my baby is getting enough (breast) milk?

Etc. etc. There was nothing – not a single sentence in the entire guide produced by UNICEF and the Department of Health and all the other members of the great and the good – about what to do if you can't manage to breastfeed.

After my week in hospital, literally just as I was leaving, I was finally handed a leaflet about bottle-feeding – not quite in a brown paper bag, but almost. Visually it was by far the poor relation to its cheerful, vibrant, breastfeeding cousin. In plain typeface and with a minimal amount of functional photographs, it explained how to make up a feed and sterilise bottles.

The advice about 'eating out' was a corker:

'If' you have to go out, it said, you must use freshly boiled water to make up your feed and it must not be lower than 70 degrees and it must be consumed within two hours.

The last two pages were, of course, dedicated to telling you that you shouldn't really be doing any of this at all.

So for the first month of my baby's life, I didn't dare venture more than ten minutes away from home and the trusty steam steriliser my husband panic-bought before picking us up from the maternity ward.

CHAPTER 3

The Science Bit

Reece and I had talked about breastfeeding, of course. We attended an entire antenatal class on the subject (yet again no mention really of the alternative. Apparently an old section on bottle-feeding has been edited out by most Primary Care Trusts).

We knew that breast equalled best.

And yet not one person (and I must by now have spoken to over 50 midwives, health visitors and breastfeeding counsellors) has ever been able to tell me about a single specific study or statistic that actually proves this.

I'm sure it's out there, so come on! Shout about it! Show me the money, as it were. Tell me about the one million breastfed babies who lived to be 150, or won *Who Wants to Be a Millionaire*, or never got colds. Yes, I could Google it, but isn't this the kind of info the health advisors should be reeling off at every given opportunity?

Surely there could have been a spare paragraph inside that lovely breastfeeding booklet with its happy pictures of smiling, fluffy babes sucking on impossibly pert, round breasts to go ever so slightly into what TV documentaries call 'the science bit'?

Personally I would really like to see more 'science bits' in the whole world of natal healthcare. When I was heavily pregnant I watched a BBC programme called *Misbehaving Mums to Be*. I don't know how the producers found their subjects, but it featured mainly very young women stroking their baby bumps while smoking fags, eating deep-fried pizzas and coming out with pearls of wisdom like 'I think smoking is good for my baby because their heart has to work harder so it means they will be stronger'.

The midwife who specialised in getting smoking mums to quit didn't seem to have much luck. Almost every week the episode ended with the mum in question deciding that it was too stressful to give up, and essentially ignoring the midwife's phone calls.

I think it was because the midwife had such a rubbish gadget to measure stuff on. The pregnant mum had to breathe into a tube and then a number would flash up onscreen next to a generic little baby silhouette slowly getting a Ready Brek glow.

The midwife would adopt a sad expression.

'You see, you're an eighteen,' she would say forlornly. 'And that's not good for baby.'

Leaving baffled viewers like me shouting, 'Eighteen WHAT? Out of HOW MANY?' at the telly in exasperation.

I reached for the cookie jar each time the bemused mother on screen went straight outside for a Silk Cut. I gave up watching when I put on half a pound after watching two episodes back to back. Not enough of a science bit, you see?

I already had my suspicions about the seemingly vague nature of my own natal care. When I was 38 weeks pregnant, I wrote this blog post about my observations up until that point:

The rules change. A lot.
The last time I saw my midwife at my local health centre she took a urine sample, tested it and then gave it back to me, saying that she couldn't dispose of it and so I had to take it home. This has never happened before (and she has done the same test each time I've seen her, in the same place, every four weeks for the last eight months). I can only conclude that I am now weeing Kryptonite and that this is somehow harmful to the people of my local community.

There's no school like the old-school
I'm convinced that antenatal classes are designed by nursery school teachers, motivational speakers and Blue Peter presenters on acid. So far I've had a pink ping-pong ball in a jam jar full of water thrust at me (apparently to represent the baby's head in the pelvis), an empty round box of cheese triangles waved around to illustrate cervical dilation

[remember that?], knitted breasts (neither my partner nor I can remember them being used, they were just there on the table, like an entertainingly perverse centrepiece at a dinner party) and a wooden box with a paddle to demonstrate the baby's path out of the womb. I've also been encouraged to 'brainstorm' the membrane, the cervix and the first stage of labour with a group of other first-time parents who were equally agog.

Oh, and halfway through you get a glass of squash and a biscuit.

The quacks are out there

A couple of weeks ago the midwife decided the baby may be breech (i.e. feet down rather than head down). Her solution was to either put a bag of frozen peas where she believed the head to be, or to contact another midwife who was trained in moxibustion. This is a practice derived from acupuncture in which herbs are burned on a pregnant woman's foot to encourage the baby to turn. The moxibustion midwife told me to 'work on my priorities' when I was unable to meet her at her **private** clinic (her NHS appointments being, of course, fully booked). This from a woman who burns people's feet for a living. A scan at the hospital revealed that happily the baby is in fact exactly where it should be. So I suppose my priorities are officially back in order.

Midwives vs hospital consultants

I have been under the care of both midwife and consultant because of a previous thyroid problem. From what I can see there is a mutual mistrust between the two. Probably not helped by the fact that the first time I saw the consultant, it turned out the midwife had not carried out the right blood tests for my thyroid condition. She blamed the hospital, the lab and even the courier before it could finally be admitted that she'd forgotten to do it, despite writing in my notes that she had.

When the midwife diagnosed breech, she told me the consultant would probably book me in for a caesarean on the spot and warned me to 'be strong', like having a c-section was a form of ritual humiliation rather than a medical alternative. The consultant cheerfully said nothing more than that she thought the midwife had confused baby's head with baby's bottom. In response the midwife now points out that the consultant still wrote 'breech' *with a question mark by it* in my maternity notes every time I see her. I think these relationship problems are all due to bad communication.

These professionals only ever see each other in the few words they scribble in the maternity notes that the patient dutifully carries around absolutely everywhere (Seriously. You'd think in this day and age it could just be a memory stick. A rainforest has quite probably vanished thanks to my ever-expanding paper folder alone). Of course they sound a bit abrupt, even aloof. *'Breech?'* doesn't exactly give you much to go on, and being surrounded by pregnant women all the time must mean their own hormones are running riot. Perhaps it's just not coming across in quite the way it was intended.

Boy did I open a can of worms with that post. I was really astonished by the comments I received – because although I hadn't even mentioned it, the people who replied were almost entirely expressing deep anger about breastfeeding support. Perhaps alarm bells should have rung at the time. But now I know why they felt so strongly about it. From the very first response:

> If there's one thing especially that's fucked up about pregnancy care is [sic] the religious approach to breastfeeding and the piling on of guilt and shame if you even dare to suggest you're moving on to the bottle. Yes, I'm quite certain it's better, evolution is good like that, but if it's destroying your sanity or worse, potentially harming your baby then stop, buy some SMA, and get on with looking after the kid. A few friends have had this problem and it makes me livid every time.

Encouragement from another (not that I knew I would need it at the time):

> As for breastfeeding – I tried for about 10 days and then said the hell with it. My son grew up to achieve a Ph.D in neuroanatomy, so I guess I didn't scar him too badly.

Wrote a third:

> Heh. 'sweet' memories. Militant midwifes, Booby-filled guilt trips... Our 21 month old was bottle all the way. The best bit of advice I can give you is, Ironically, ignore any advice from anyone else, especially post-natal midwives. We had 3 midwives. one said we shouldn't give (our baby) water as well as formula, one said we should and the other said it didn't make any difference. Like 3 wise monkeys. More like wise-arse donkeys.

And:

> I remember that in the maternity hospital, they posted up a flowchart of what to expect when you ask for formula milk for your baby. And it seriously included the immortal phrase 'Health worker to remind mother of the benefits of breast milk'.

And so on.

Okay, there's no science bit there either. But there is a whole lot of anger and guilt. Surely that's not supposed to be your very first introduction to parenthood?

CHAPTER 4

Bosom Bother

In the run-up to the birth Reece and I were very relaxed about breastfeeding. We casually decided that we would give it a go, and if it didn't work out, so be it. That said, we had no back-up plan either.

I now think we were blasé about it because it genuinely didn't occur to us that it wouldn't happen. We're both educated people and it's a pretty basic instinct, right? Baby knows where the food is and mother knows to make it.

It's telling that in the run-up to Harrison's birth neither of us bought a steriliser, bottles, formula. But we did buy nipple cream, nipple pads and breast milk storage bags. For months afterwards they looked at me sadly from the top of the bathroom cabinet because even once I knew for sure that it wasn't going to happen, I couldn't throw them away just in case it suddenly did. Even a year later I still got the odd drop of milk if I squeezed my breasts really hard – but even at my peak, as it were, I rarely got much more than that. In the end I sold the pads and milk bags for £1 at a jumble sale. A friend got the nipple cream. At least they helped others, I suppose.

Millions of years of evolution have gone into perfecting breastfeeding techniques. I've watched countless mammals do it on teatime wildlife programmes. Kate Humble never showed off a newborn with nipple confusion on *Lambing Live*. How hard can it be? If you can master a street-dance fitness class (okay, I wasn't particularly great at those either), surely you can get the hang of baby-meets-boob pretty quickly. That's what I thought.

So when Harrison was born and in my arms, the first thing I thought I should do was feed him. Weighing just shy of six pounds, while he wasn't technically underweight, he was definitely in need of a decent meal. He lay on my chest and I waited for him to do 'the crawl', this strange little routine that newborns apparently do as they root around looking for your breast. He didn't.

'It's okay,' soothed the midwife. 'It can take up to twelve hours for them to have their first feed. You both need to rest.'

So Harrison went into a cot and she ran me a bath.

I am a bath snob. I am on a lifelong pilgrimage of the world's best places in which to float around in warm water. On our wedding night Reece and I languished in a giant, sunken corner bath in the bridal suite of our luxury hotel for nearly two hours. I've swum through the winter mist at night in an outdoor hot spa in Iceland and wallowed in an ornate, tenth-century, underground natural pool far beneath Budapest.

This is partly why I don't like our bath at home. I've been spoiled. I'd rather have a cold shower than a disappointing bath. But I can honestly say that the bath I took after giving birth, in a narrow NHS tub under strip lighting with no bath foam (I wasn't allowed), was the best soak I have ever had.

Unfortunately my blissful, post-bath inner calm had completely dissipated by midday the following day when Harrison was 12 hours old and still showed no interest in the whole 'crawl' business. So the midwife decided to put him on my breast herself.

When you see pictures of babies breastfeeding, they look angelic. Little, pink, round cheeks, shiny-eyed with contentment and a mouth full of boob.

Our baby looked nothing like that. When faced with my boobs, he would pull the same face I would after sucking several very bitter lemons. Then he would jerk his head away and scream until he was bright red, his little gums flashing angrily as the midwife repeatedly grabbed hold of the back of his neck and forced his head down onto my chest. I was shocked by the way he was manhandled and I can't begin to tell you how much the rejection stung. It simply had not occurred to me that he wouldn't be up for it. Why wasn't he up for it? I suppose I'll never know – although I later found out from my own mother that I was the same.

After a tortuous 25 minutes of this it was decided that I would 'express' instead. At that point I wasn't really producing much in the way of milk. The very first milk, called colostrum, is 'rocket fuel', said the midwife, and the baby didn't need much. Which was just as well, as another 30 minutes was then agonisingly and humiliatingly spent massaging and squeezing tiny droplets of the stuff from my breasts and collecting them into a small syringe. There was less than a millilitre in the tube by the end. The midwife told me this was the part of the job they all hated doing. Thanks for that.

I felt like a complete failure. My breasts had never been a disappointment before – I would even go so far as to say that they had traditionally been a bit of an asset, and they looked pretty good in a decent bra. Now they felt sore and useless. Harrison was tiny and needed me, and on his first day in the world I had let him down.

'We'll try him again in three hours,' said the midwife as she left. That set the pattern – every three hours, night and day, for the duration of my stay a midwife would come in, wake us up if necessary and attempt a feed.

I can't remember whether Reece was there or not that first time. He probably was as he rarely left my side until late at night – partners were only allowed to stay over during labour – but I felt so alone and tearful. And I was already dreading the next attempt.

It was the same story three hours later. And again three hours after that. Harrison would not try to latch on to my nipples and my milk supply was minimal to say the least. I could not understand it. At work I had once interviewed a woman who regularly donated her breast milk to hospitals because she produced so much. She had a freezer full of the stuff, all labelled up in little bags. So where the hell was mine?

That night the midwives began to grow concerned. A blood test revealed that Harrison's blood sugars were low and he was wheezing a little. Reluctantly a paediatrician was summoned.

'In an ideal world you want to avoid the paediatricians at all costs,' the midwife told me through gritted teeth in a way that made me feel strangely guilty. It reminded me once more of my now-weirdly-prescient blog post in which I'd suggested that doctors and midwives didn't appear to be great friends.

The paediatrician, a Nordic woman with a crisp accent, took one look at my son and said, 'This baby is extremely hungry. He needs to eat – now.'

I could practically hear the proverbial heckles rising on the midwife's back.

'He's had expressed colostrum,' she said stiffly.

When the doctor heard about the miniscule amounts he had been given, she snorted and addressed me for the first time.

'He needs some formula,' she said. 'SMA or Cow & Gate?'

CHAPTER 5

Slippery Slopes

Up until this point all the midwives had been waxing lyrical about Day Three. Three days after you give birth you wake up with tits like Pamela Anderson, they told me. These rock-hard gigantabreasts would literally appear overnight and I would suddenly start spurting milk like a lactating Trevi fountain (one mum told me her partner found it so arousing when it happened that from then on she sprayed him with milk whenever they shagged. Each to their own). This would all be possible because Day Three is when the milk 'comes in'. Hallelujah.

We can cope with the formula thing until then, I thought. After all, he was only having ten millilitres at a time (that's only half a shot glass) and he was being made to sip it from a cup in order to avoid the dreaded 'nipple confusion'. To be honest he was so hungry I think he'd have figured out a way to pull it out of my hair if he'd had to.

Surely Harrison wouldn't lose out on his future membership of Mensa because of a few droplets of artificial milk? Apparently some study or other 'indicated' that breastfed babies have a higher IQ by 8.9 points than bottle-fed babies. Mind you, when I grew up being left-handed was considered a disability and guess what? That too was linked to formula-feeding. It seems there is almost nothing formula can't fuck up, if you spend long enough Googling it.

Anyway, back to the much-anticipated Day Three. Almost as an aside, the midwives mentioned that I would also feel like complete shit, because as well as Milk Moment, Day Three is also Baby Blues Day. That's because your hormones go on the rampage and you pretty much cry the whole time. But who cares, was the undertone, because you can breastfeed! And you also get to look like Pamela Anderson. What more do you want?

I only had 24 hours to go.

The morning midwife was livid about the formula incident. I'd 'ruined the baby's stomach lining', she told me, and I was 'on a slippery slope'. That sounded ominous, even though she never enlightened me as to which slope this was or why it was so highly polished. It was as if not only had I somehow deliberately chosen to not produce enough breast milk, but I'd also destroyed my baby's life by listening to the doctor. It struck me once more that doctors and midwives really need to learn how to get along. The staff Christmas do must be painful.

Now I come to think of it (at the time I was too tired and emotional to do anything more intellectual than cry. A lot.) that culture clash reminds me of a story I heard from a formula-feeding mum who had her first child in the Midlands in the 1970s. A doctor came to see her, took one look at her and, without asking her any questions, said, 'With a bosom like yours, you should be breastfeeding,' before promptly discharging her. Meanwhile, in another hospital further north, one of my friends had also just been born and her mother, along with the rest of her ward, was given Epsom salts to dry up her milk because breastfeeding was considered dirty. Right hand, meet left hand... It's been going on for years.

Back on my ward in 2011, the fact that Harrison's blood sugars were back to normal again and he was both calm and content for the first time in his short life apparently wasn't worth mentioning.

I now know I was lucky to get anything at all. Birmingham Women's Hospital stopped providing formula milk 'except in emergencies' on 1 July 2011 and the policy had already been introduced in nearby Walsall by then. Google 'NHS' and 'formula-feed' and you'll find it popping up as a discussion thread on various parenting message boards with mums reporting that they are increasingly expected to 'bring their own bottles' in hospitals across the country from Dewsbury to south Essex.

The nature of the conversations can generally be summarised as either 'If you don't breastfeed, you deserve everything you get' or 'Whatever happened to freedom of choice?'.

You can guess which sort appealed more to me, especially as had I been in Birmingham or Dewsbury both my son and I would have been completely screwed. Even if I had known where to score formula milk at 4 a.m. on a Wednesday morning, I had stitches in places that never saw daylight and I had not yet managed to walk ten metres down the corridor to the communal kitchen for a cup of tea, let alone stagger a mile down the road to the nearest 24-hour store and hit the shops. It wouldn't surprise me if there were some kind of licensing laws surrounding the stuff. No Smirnoff or SMA after 11 p.m.

Mind you, hospitals don't provide nappies any more either, I suppose – and as far as I'm aware, even breastfed babies need those. I had to bring my own bath towel too. Times are indeed tough, but I'd still rather go without a shower than see a baby go without food.

Day Two had not got off to a great start.

CHAPTER 6

Judgement Day

If Day Two was bad then Day Three was even worse. I woke up tearful, exhausted and with no sign of the promised porn star boobs. Every time a new midwife came on shift and popped her head around the door I found myself having to explain the situation all over again and was met with varying degrees of disapproval over the F-word.

As time went on whenever I explained about my lack of milk to midwives then health visitors then other so-called experts, they would almost always reply 'Don't feel bad' without my saying that I did in a way that made me feel instantly miserable. I am by nature a people-pleaser and I couldn't shake the knowledge that I was – and still am – being judged.

They almost always referred to the formula-feeding as 'my choice', which made me want to howl because it wasn't my choice at all but the cards I had been dealt. What choice did I actually have? Feed my baby with the food I could provide and follow the doctor's advice, or play the waiting game and take a gamble that my milk would decide to turn up before the baby got really ill.

Now, my husband takes angrily to social network platform Twitter whenever an advert for formula milk comes on the telly and goes on about breast being best. But in the words of one, *'If you decide to move on...'* then such-and-such a brand is the one for you. What about all of us for whom there is no choice? And actually, fuck it, even if it is your choice, why should society beat you up about it?

The only reason I spent a whole week in hospital was because I was strongly advised to stay until breastfeeding was 'established'. Towards the end it began to feel like they might as well have told me to stay there until I became six feet tall.

Talk about waiting for Godot.

Anyway, back to Day Three. At this point the best way to describe our breastfeeding technique was an absolute fucking mess. Harrison and I were not natural dining companions. If we'd been on a dinner date I'd have accidentally spilled my soup in his lap and he would have had a violent allergic reaction to the chicken satay.

As his conversation skills were limited, he did the only thing he knew how to do – he screamed blue murder every time his head was forced onto my boob by various midwives every three hours. After up to half an hour of that, these same midwives would then wring a few drops out of me by massaging and squeezing my breasts for as long as it took – sometimes there would be less than an hour before the whole process had to start again. I am quite sure he dreaded the whole thing as much as I did. For me, it was utterly mortifying, painful and frustrating.

Boy did I need those boobs to hurry up and get here.

My husband Reece had just about managed to convince me that I wasn't poisoning Harrison with the formula milk and that actually it was the only solution given the circumstances when a 'breastfeeding counsellor' decided to pay us a visit.

What I got was as far from any form of counselling as it's possible to get. In fact, I have since considered getting counselling to deal with the counselling that I didn't have, bonkers as that sounds.

This counsellor and I didn't discuss whether there was any reason that I may have problems with breastfeeding (retired midwifery lecturer Sue Battersby later told me women who have been sexually abused, for example, often can't breastfeed for psychological reasons, and while fortunately I am not one of them, according to the World Health Organization, one in five women is) or indeed how I felt about the whole thing.

In fact, nobody ever sat down with me and wondered aloud why things were not going smoothly. A friend of mine said she had heard somewhere that thyroid problems can affect milk production. In 2010, I had a benign lump removed from my neck – and half my thyroid went along with it. While the remaining half seems to be coping admirably, my thyroid hormone levels are at the bottom end of the so-called normal range.

Could this be the reason why I never lactated like mad?

Much later I emailed the UK Drugs in Lactation Advisory Service, which is there for the medical profession rather than schmucks like me, but they kindly replied anyway and told me they have 'standard texts on breastfeeding and these indicate that hypothyroidism and hyperthyroidism can affect milk production'.

However, John Lazarus, Emeritus Professor at Cardiff University School of Medicine and ex-president of the British Thyroid Association, wasn't so sure when I spoke to him.

'It wouldn't have been an issue unless you became significantly hypothyroid,' he said. 'And in that situation you would be taking thyroid tablets.'

Well, I wasn't, so perhaps that was another dead end. But look at the effort I had to go to in order to find that out for myself. No health professional who was actually supposed to be looking after me knew the first thing about it when I asked them.

Anyway, even if I had been drowning in my own milk, there was still the snag that Harrison was not remotely keen on latching on.

One of the most common problems which prevent babies latching on to the breast is tongue-tie, when the bottom of their tongue is attached to their lower mouth. Three midwives assured me that Harrison didn't have it, but a fourth one said he did and snipped the tie. She promised me it was no worse than trimming a toenail, and when she brandished the long scissors it was yet another occasion when I got far more upset about it than Harrison did. It didn't make much difference, though, so I suppose I'll never know who was right.

Back to the counsellor – she didn't even bother looking through the notes at the end of my bed, so I went through the story once again. Baby and breasts essentially not friends. In fact, baby and breasts more like Dick Dastardly in endless pursuit of that damned pigeon (you can thank my husband for that '80s cartoon reference if indeed you got it. *Wacky Races*? Oh never mind).

The counsellor's conclusion – to paraphrase – was that while I was busy having illicit encounters with the formula my breasts were doing the equivalent of taking the scissors to my most expensive clothes and throwing them out of the window.

As long as my dalliance with the little bottles continued, there would be no milk. End of. Harrison would be fine on breast milk alone and only then would more arrive, she promised. Supply and demand, and all that.

It kind of made sense. So my husband and I agreed to lay off the formula for the day. Really alarm bells should have rung when we mentioned how small he was and she basically told us that size didn't matter. I don't know a single woman who has said *that* and meant it in any other context.

You know how people sometimes repeat stuff parrot-style and you wonder whether they've really thought it through? Normally I'm quite tuned in to that sort of thing – I've worked as a journalist for so long that usually I challenge everything I'm told, which drives my family and friends nuts. But I felt a long way from the newsroom and I was too obsessed with my own breasts to think about the bigger picture. Error.

Anyway. We agreed and she left cheerfully.

Late afternoon, my mother drove down from London to see us. Our families had promised to stay away for the first two weeks but she couldn't resist, and to be honest by then I felt like a little girl lost and I wanted my own mum. So although I tutted down the phone at her, I was secretly relieved. Especially as, once I'd explained our predicament, she told me she'd been through the exact same breastfeeding nightmare with me, 33 years ago.

But when she saw Harrison she couldn't hide her shock.

'He looks..... desperate,' she blurted out, ever the diplomat.

So there I was on Day Three, all hormones and no boobs and even my own mother thought I was a parental disaster. That was how I read it anyway. I wept hysterically on the shoulder of my stunned husband. Talk about a rock and a hard place – caught bang in the middle between the wife and the mother-in-law. I'm surprised all four of us didn't spontaneously combust in a technicoloured shower of Les Dawson gags.

Needless to say, the next midwife to come on shift – yet another new face requiring a summary of our story so far – was shocked to hear that Harrison had consumed just a few drops of wrung-out breast milk all day. The entire ward was a continuity editor's nightmare – no two people seemed to share the same opinion and the conflicting advice we got from each new shift was utterly bewildering. We just couldn't win, and more importantly, guess what – Harrison's blood sugars had taken a tumble once more.

So formula was temporarily taken back off the naughty step, and a new contraption appeared:

The Breast Pump.

This little machine at least meant that I no longer had to be 'milked' by various midwives – the only thing we all agreed on was that this was a relief – and instead I could hook myself up to this electric pump which rhythmically sucked droplets of milk into a bottle that I could then give to Harrison in a cup. Except there was never enough for a cup really. Forget half-full or half-empty; this was more the dregs of the teapot. Twenty minutes each side, after a twenty-minute attempt at breastfeeding, followed by a formula 'top-up'.

There really weren't enough hours in the day. Or night.

It sounded like a life-support machine – it literally 'breathed'. After 20 minutes my nipples ached and had literally been stretched to three times their usual length. I hated it and I still don't think I'll ever be able to visit a dairy farm again. I have never felt so bovine in my life. It was, however, 'practically guaranteed' to increase my milk supply and that alone kept me going.

It didn't, of course – and we never saw that 'breastfeeding counsellor' again. Which was a shame because I have a few things I would like to say to her.

CHAPTER 7

Cuckoo's Nest

If Day Five – a Saturday – was a movie, it started out like *Mary Poppins*. Of all the midwives I met there are maybe three who were so amazing I wish I could have brought them home with me – if there weren't laws about that sort of thing.

When I was a teenager I fantasised about marrying George Michael (obviously I now know why that would never have worked out). It was less about the hot sex we would have and more about the fabulous parties we would throw with all our famous friends.

My fantasising clearly hasn't improved much in the last 20 years, because I found myself daydreaming about living with those midwives, not in a Charlie Sheen-harem type arrangement, but in some kind of idyllic birthing commune in a country home.

When I was pregnant a friend gave me a book by an American midwife called Ina May Gaskin. She runs just such a place called The Farm where pregnant women and new mums live in groups with midwives nearby. They call their homes hutches.

Okay, I'm not really into the whole 'hutch' thing. I also never managed to 'soar' through my contractions like Ina May suggested. But I still like the idea of that commune. There's safety in numbers, and you never know when you'll need it, as I was soon to discover.

I'm sitting here right now on my own with Harrison curled up like a frog on my belly, fast asleep, and I would really like to talk to those midwives. The one that sat with me in the wee hours when Harrison wouldn't sleep and told me about her family life and her dreams in her lilting Welsh voice while we soothed him.

And the other one, who was the only one who ever managed to get him to breastfeed.

She was on duty on Day Five. I don't know what it was about her, but both Harrison and I were completely smitten. She handed him to me gently and for the first time ever he latched on by himself without tears and actually stayed there on my boob for 45 minutes. She sat with me the whole time, while I tried not to shake and hardly dared to breathe in case I ruined the magical moment. He did that twice on her watch. Even though I still didn't seem to be producing much milk, there must have been something there for him to persevere for so long. I could have married her instantly.

She even returned at the end of her shift to help me again, but we were only halfway through the three-hour window between feeds and Harrison was deeply asleep. I will always regret not disturbing him. As she left she said something which, with hindsight, was a pretty bloody obvious coded warning:

'I'll try to make sure you get a nice midwife tonight.'

I remember thinking it was a bit of an odd thing to say. But of the midwives I'd met so far, some were undeniably nicer than others, and she was at that point the best adult I'd ever met in my life. So I dismissed it and decided to grab an hour of much-needed sleep, happy in the knowledge that we had finally cracked this breast bother.

At this point the movie that was Day Five changed from *Mary Poppins* to *One Flew Over the Cuckoo's Nest*. If there was a celestial projectionist in charge of the film reels that day, I hope he, she or it was fired.

I was awoken by the sound of the woman in the room next door being dragged to hell by the hair – or having the noisiest labour I have ever heard. Her agonised howls reverberated around my room as if she was in bed next to me, and in between contractions I heard her whimper 'Just a minute, just a minute.' But of course there never was just a minute, and soon she was off once again.

I opened my eyes. In his clear cot next to me, I could see Harrison was awake too. His eyes twinkled in the darkness but he didn't cry. We just looked at each other.

Then our little bonding moment was exposed in a glare of strip lighting as the night shift midwife came in to help with his next feed.

She didn't seem particularly happy about it and I suddenly felt like the last thing I wanted to do in front of this woman was get my boobs out. But that was why she was there, so I gritted my teeth and stripped off my nightie while she manhandled Harrison out of his cot. I remember thinking that it looked like she was holding him by the scruff of the neck as she thrust his face onto my left breast.

To try to make conversation I asked her whether the woman in labour was doing okay. I know, not the best ice breaker because she clearly wasn't – but it was the only thing that sprung to mind and the midwife may have been eye to eye with my boobs but she didn't look like she was about to ask me about my holiday plans any time soon.

'I don't know, not my room,' she replied tartly.

Harrison by this point was already crimson and giving the woman next door a run for her money. The midwife tutted and pushed him even harder, trying to jam my nipple in his mouth, which by now was wide open and screaming.

'How premature was he?' she demanded as he wriggled furiously in her grasp and howled. I could see red finger marks on his neck and between his shoulders and I was about to protest but the question stopped me in my tracks. Nobody had used that word before.

'Um, he was only two days early,' I said shakily, thinking perhaps I had misheard.

She shook her head. 'They must have got the dates wrong. What did they say at your scans?'

I bit back my tears. 'They said he was due on the twenty-third of June,' I whispered.

'How about the midwife? Did you have regular measurements from her?'

I couldn't believe this was happening. What was she getting at and why was she channelling Nurse Ratched from *One Flew Over the Cuckoo's Nest*?

'Yes, I saw her every month and she measured my uterus...'

When you're pregnant your uterus grows by one centimetre a week. So when you're 20 weeks gone your uterus is 20 centimetres long from your pelvis up towards your stomach, and on it goes.

However, this apparently wasn't a reliable enough method of marking time.

'What?!' she snorted. 'I mean... how long is a piece of string? Why didn't you ask her to do it properly?'

I had no idea what she was talking about. There had never been any suggestion that this uterus-measuring method was inaccurate or unprofessional (and even now, to my knowledge, it isn't) or that there were other alternatives.

'Because, you evil old cow, I've never done this before!' is what I should have said. And in any case I knew exactly when Harrison had been conceived. It simply wasn't biologically possible for the dates to be wrong.

Instead, tired, emotional and feeling more vulnerable than I ever have in my entire life, I said: 'I don't know... Do you think he's premature then?'

'Oh yes,' she said, I swear with a hint of triumph. 'You can tell by the way he's behaving.'

Poor Harrison was still thrashing about under her iron grip. I secretly hoped he would give her a kick but if he did I feared she would throw him out of the window.

And then she played her trump card:

'You haven't cooked this one properly.'

Ouch. Somehow I managed to pull myself together enough to say that I thought we were done with the breastfeeding attempt and could I please have some formula now? (I wasn't allowed to keep it in my room, for some spurious health and safety reason, I believe. Each time a new bottle had to be bought in, maybe in case I somehow accidentally overdosed on it like paracetamol).

She thrust Harrison into my arms and swept away. At the door she turned around and announced: 'The next feed will be three hours from the start of this last one.' Until now Harrison's feeding pattern had been every three hours from the *end* of the last feed, and the duty midwife would come in to help. This change pretty much meant that by the time I'd finished expressing she'd be back.

Harrison and I were both shaking. He was hysterical and I felt like the doomed heroine in a horror movie.

I'm in bedlam, I thought as the woman next door's wails echoed around the room (Harrison by this point was so apoplectic he was no longer making a noise, just open-mouthed in one huge, silent Edvard Munchian scream). *I've somehow been sectioned in this Dickensian asylum and I'm never, ever going to get out of here.*

I hate that word – cooked. Firstly no woman is an oven, and secondly the suggestion, beyond a shadow of a doubt, was that it was all my fault. Like that time when I was heavily pregnant and I made chocolate muffins but used the wrong flour by mistake. They were more like oversized soft biscuits than anything that could possibly be described as cake-like.

Now that I can hold my hands up to. The development of an embryo, however, is a trickier to control. I didn't smoke or drink or take any class As, Bs or Cs. I didn't eat pâté and I took my folic acid every day (well, almost). I'd followed the bloody recipe to the letter – hadn't I?

I cast my mind back over the last 40 weeks. Where had I gone wrong? In the first couple of weeks, before I knew I was expecting, I'd drunk a bit of wine with friends. Had the little DNA helix that told Harrison how to breastfeed got too hammered to pass on the message? Woken up the next morning with a thumping headache and a nagging feeling that it had forgotten something important?

Also, I hadn't quit the local running club until week 12. Had I pounded all my milk ducts into the residential streets around which we leisurely jogged every Wednesday night after work?

Once you start going down this path of mental torture it's difficult to change tack. Fortunately Harrison came to my rescue by doing a very loud, very aromatic newborn poo.

As I changed his nappy I contemplated keeping the old one as a weapon to use against the evil midwife if she returned. But that probably would have got me sectioned for real.

I debated putting a chair against the door and sleeping with one eye open just in case, but she must have moved on to her next victim because another nurse came in to do the next feed. I tearfully told her I did not want to see the evil midwife again. She had traumatised my baby, I said (*and me*, I added silently).

Premature? Really? It still haunts me, despite everybody I've asked since assuring me that he was not. He certainly has none of the discernible health problems that premature babies can be prone to.

I texted Reece.

Fucking evil midwife on tonight. She practically broke Harrison's neck forcing him onto my breast and went on to me about thinking he's 'not cooked properly'...

His reply:

Tell her to piss off from me. He's perfect. Why does all this happen when I'm not there? So frustrating...

Good point, I thought. I bet she wouldn't have done it if there had been any more reliable witnesses in the room than a five-day-old baby and his mad, hormonal, sleep-deprived mum.

I think I'm going to have to just manage through the night on my own, I replied. It was the first time I'd even thought about trying to cope by myself. I didn't feel ready – but I couldn't bear the alternative.

I'm not going to go through that again. He was purple with screaming – worst ever. I just hope it doesn't put us back to square one. (Obviously I can't prove that it did, but Harrison never breastfed from me again like he had done earlier that day.)

You don't want her touching you, wrote Reece. *We are leaving tomorrow when I get there.*

CHAPTER 8

The Great Escape

Reece came storming into the hospital the next morning on a huge white steed, brandishing a sword and shield emblazoned with a crest featuring an elaborate milk bottle. He whisked me and Harrison straight out of my NHS bed and onto the back of the rearing stallion, and together we leapt through the window and rode off into the horizon, my long, blonde locks streaming behind me.

Did I mention that I hadn't had much sleep back then? My hair hasn't grown below my shoulders in years and as far as I'm aware they don't let horses into maternity wards these days. I may have accidentally given birth on the biblical essence of frankincense rather than the more conventional pethidine, but even I know I wasn't anywhere near any stables.

The night shift had finished, meaning Nurse Ratched was no longer on the prowl. I think if Reece had seen her it would have been more than Harrison's nappy that went flying across the room. Reece informed the next midwife we saw that unless there was any medical reason for us to stay, we were leaving.

The atmosphere seemed to change immediately.

In that case, said the midwife, she would ask a paediatrician to come and see us with a feeding plan.

And that was it.

When I was in my twenties my best friend and I would weigh up social invitations on the basis of how easy it was to leave if the soirée (for it was almost always an evening bash) turned out to be a bit shit. Needless to say, we would never have accepted an invite to this one – and yet it wasn't so hard to make our excuses and bugger off after all.

Remember *Red Dwarf*? Cult British sci-fi book by Rob Grant and Doug

Naylor which ended up being a TV series? I didn't watch the series but I devoured the books (I accidentally told Craig Charles this once when I found myself out drinking with him and some mutual friends. He played the main character in the TV show. Well, how was I to know?).

In one of the books – and no doubt one of the TV episodes too (that was for you, Craig) – the characters get stuck in a virtual world (it was way ahead of its time there, written long before the days of *World of Warcraft* and *Second Life*).

That world was a game called *Better Than Life* and it was fatal because you had such a good time there you forgot about the real world and you ended up dying because you weren't looking after your actual self. There were all these emergency exit signs in the game that you could walk through to wake up, but nobody did because they were having such fun they'd forgotten it wasn't real.

I was a long way from having the time of my life, but I too had completely forgotten that I was free to go. I had been told so often that I should stay until I had 'established' breastfeeding, it had totally slipped my mind that I had a choice... and I certainly hadn't been reminded.

But that was it – as soon as Reece uttered the magic words 'We're leaving' it was as if something finally clicked into gear. Instead of pacing around in my room singing Beatles songs to Harrison and waiting for my boobs to channel Lolo Ferrari, it was time at last for the staff to tell us something useful, like how the hell to look after our gorgeous little boy in our own home.

A paediatrician dropped by and gave us more practical advice in ten minutes than we had heard all week. He confirmed what I had believed all along: that the pathetic mouthfuls of breast milk I was producing were not enough to nurture a newborn. Not one of the midwives had been able or willing to quantify for me how much was enough (because it's organic, you see, it doesn't come out in convenient measurements) but he finally did, and essentially it turned out I was supplying less than a fifth of the volume Harrison needed to feel full. And his stomach was only the size of a marble. So that really was pretty lame.

Imagine going to a dinner party, having eaten nothing all day in preparation, only to find that the main (and only) course is half a salmon blini. You'd be pretty pissed off, and more importantly mentally planning an immediate escape to the nearest late-night cafe. I guess in my son's case, that was the formula-feed.

Still, we were only allowed to give it to him from a cup in case, God forbid, he actually started enjoying it. Harrison wasn't even a week old and he'd barely had a single meal that wasn't a complete misery. I found myself wondering at what point he'd give up on it altogether and stop eating at all. I know I would have done – I'm a stubborn cow like that and he has at least half of my obstinate DNA.

So the paediatrician gave us his plan. Thirty millilitres of formula every three hours topped up with whatever I could express. Simples. It meant I would still be expressing an awful lot, but at least I'd be comfortable on my own sofa.

Reece legged it into town to buy all the formula-related paraphernalia we hadn't bothered to get before Harrison was born.

Needless to say no one could or would give us any advice about recommended brands, or the best sort of steriliser. (This in itself is a whole new world. The bottle steriliser market is surprisingly lucrative, it turns out. You can steam, soak or heat your way to hygiene using a bucket, a microwave or any number of specially designed electric gadgets. None of them come cheap. By the way you should not, as one midwife suggested to a mum I know, use the dishwasher.)

One of the midwives showed us how to make up the formula (apparently not many hospitals even do this much), Harrison and I were both given a quick once-over and that was it, we were free to go. All that remained was to figure out how the fuck the seat belt was going to fit around our brand new infant car seat, but by that point frankly I could more easily have learned quantum physics than listened to any more well-intentioned advice about breastfeeding.

As we were leaving I asked two of the midwives who had looked after me before whether they had found breastfeeding as hard as I had. One told me she had no problems but gave up after six weeks when a growth spurt meant that her baby was constantly attached to a boob, and the other said she had only breastfed one of her children and didn't say why.

I felt betrayed. These two had been so persuasive and encouraging that I should persevere and sit tight and do the Lambada in order to get my milk to appear – and unbeknownst to me, it hadn't worked out for them either. So much for the bloody sisterhood. I wonder now how they must have felt about doing that. Perhaps they thought they were doing me a favour, or felt gagged by their profession. Or maybe it was just another shift on the rota and they didn't feel anything at all.

It was the first inkling I had that we women are really not helping each other out here. Look up 'breastfeeding problems' online and you'll find millions of us proudly stating that we ate cow dung and drank ammonia for six months but IT WORKED and little Tarquin/Destiny/Fifilulu happily breastfed until the age of nine.

I have one plea, ladies. Can we please stop this right now? This one-upmanship, this refusal to accept that for some women it just doesn't happen? Not so long ago a woman whispered to me the horrifying news that she knew of a health visitor who was ANTI-BREASTFEEDING. She said it in the same way one might describe a person as being an axe murderer.

'Apparently she goes into people's homes, and if they're having problems with breastfeeding, she just tells them to GO ON THE BOTTLE!' she kvetched, like the woman was condoning a healthy dose of cyanide before bedtime.

I don't know who that health visitor is, but whoever you are, lady, I salute you. Thank you for being the voice of reason. In your honour, from now on every time I see an online forum thread that begins 'I am having an absolute nightmare...' I'm going to incur the wrath of the masses and use the f-word. FORMULA. There, I said it.

Yeah.

That felt good.

CHAPTER 9

The Breast Whisperer

Close one door and another opens, the saying goes. The next morning I opened mine to find another bloody midwife on the driveway.

I had been up most of the night and it's no exaggeration to say I looked like shit. Gone was the polished journalist who presented herself, immaculately dressed, at all the routine pre-baby checkups. In her place was a bleary-eyed, tearful new mum with greasy hair and baby sick on her pyjamas. It was the anti-makeover. Gok Wan would have had a heart attack.

Still, if it hadn't been for the baby sick I would have hugged her because she was the midwife I had seen for the last nine months. A familiar face and, I hoped, not a judgemental one.

We discussed breastfeeding and I showed her the drama we went through at feeding time and the small amount of milk I seemed to be producing (I had continued the three-hourly expressing routine overnight and by hand because I was still determined that the formula was only a 'top-up', even though the reality was that it was very much the main course). If you ever want to contemplate the futility of existence, try sitting in your lounge at 4 a.m. squeezing drops of milk from your own boobs into a tiny cup for 40 minutes at a time. Character building it ain't.

The midwife had the solution, however. What I needed (apart from a sanity check and 24 hours of uninterrupted sleep) was a lady Reece christened The Breast Whisperer. This woman, the lactational Derren Brown of our small town, was guaranteed to get my juices flowing, as it were.

So the next morning she arrived, bearing yet another electric breast pump. All that was missing was a little wooden stall and a farmer's daughter.

Harrison was asleep in the bedroom with my husband when The Breast Whisperer turned up, so I asked her to wait in the lounge while I fetched him.

Instead she followed me right in and bade a cheerful 'Good morning' to my bewildered, stark-bollock-naked other half as I lifted Harrison from his Moses basket and tried to pretend this was a perfectly normal situation for us all to be in.

She then followed me through to the kitchen and started barking at me for preparing Harrison's formula wrong and not making enough. I explained that we were following the advice of the hospital paediatrician (she practically crossed herself on hearing that word), but apparently either he was talking out of his arse or I hadn't listened properly.

I am renowned among my friends for not taking any shit. A few years ago I lived with two good friends in London and whenever we had problems with the letting agent I was sent in as a last resort because I was by far the most ferocious. (We had problems ridiculously regularly. On the day we moved in the place hadn't been cleaned. Then there was the time we were without a fridge in the height of summer for three weeks... but I digress).

Wherever this 'old' me had been hiding, she finally burst through the door and I found myself telling The Breast Whisperer that if she was going to follow me around my own home criticising my every move then I would have to ask her to leave (or words to that effect). It felt so good – for me, if not for The Breast Whisperer, who I expect was not very accustomed to being challenged by exhausted new mums in blue satin pyjamas – especially, as my husband fondly says, since those pyjamas make me look like a giant Quality Street.

She changed tack pretty quickly.

I'm not sure what magical solution I expected her to have to my milk draught drama, but once we'd run through the usual ('Have you tried holding the baby under your arm like a bowling ball?') we were left with relying on the pump to get things going. Yup, the same thing that hadn't worked in the hospital, but hey, let's persevere anyway. At this point the phrases 'flogging' and 'dead horse' would probably have sprung to mind had I not been far too shattered to attempt anything as clever as word association.

I later found out that The Breast Whisperer actually rang the hospital after she left us to check on the advice we had been given. So much for patient confidentiality, not to mention basic trust.

And guess what? The pump didn't work. The only thing it did was to make me feel increasingly alienated from my family. One afternoon I was sitting on the sofa attached to it as per usual while I watched Reece play with Harrison on his little baby gym. I felt like I was watching a family scene on the telly rather than watching my own. When I told Reece he said I should play with Harrison more myself. I went mental. 'When the f-u-c-k [yup, I spelled it out] do I have time to do that?!' I screamed. Anyone would think that parenthood was supposed to be FUN.

After a fortnight of this we finally made the decision to 'give up'. I never saw The Breast Whisperer again (now I come to think of it, I believe I still owe her a tenner for the pump hire. Oops) and we got on with bottle-feeding our baby. I stopped the three-hourly expressing following the inevitable frustrated tantrum that Harrison threw every time we tried to get him to latch on.

Two weeks after that I was lying in bed with him next to me. He randomly moved towards me, latched on and stayed there for an hour. I was absolutely gobsmacked.

My milk never did 'come in' as far as I'm aware (no giant boobs, no sexy milk fountains), and Harrison continued to bottle-feed. He would breastfeed when he wanted to and I'm pretty sure I was always more of an hors d'oeuvre than a Sunday roast, or maybe just a living, breathing pacifier, but it wasn't until we both relaxed about it and moved away from the ridiculous pressure put upon us by the so-called professionals that we even got started.

I can't tell you how angry that makes me feel.

CHAPTER 10

Education, Education, Education

In the first two weeks of Harrison's life I'd received so much conflicting information about pretty much every aspect of feeding him that I was rapidly coming to the conclusion that not only did the proverbial left hand not know what the right hand was doing, but it didn't even know there was a right hand. Or any other body part for that matter.

After 37 years as a midwife and midwifery lecturer, Dr Sue Battersby has now retired, but in 2009 she carried out some research into midwives' knowledge and understanding of bottle-feeding.

She interviewed 110 midwives around the country. She found that two-thirds of them did not 'normally' provide information about formula and even more did not know anything about the different brands.

'I think a lot of feeds aren't made up correctly,' Dr Battersby told me. 'Midwives give out wrong instructions because they have very limited instructions themselves about formula-feed. It is a dilemma – how do you improve midwives' knowledge so they can be more informative without being academic and going over the mother's head?'

As I've said already, personally I'd have preferred a bit of academia. Starting with some cold, hard facts. Midwifery is now a university degree subject after all, and frankly I'd rather be the one to make the decision about which information is 'over my head'. I can be a right pain in the arse about things like that – but I realise not everyone is as dogged as me.

But then Dr Battersby said something that concerned me even more: 'When the Department of Health issues new recommendations they are often not passed down to the midwives – there are very few forums to enable them to do that.'

We all know how easy it is to ignore the company newsletters and all-staff emails that flutter into your inbox when you least want them – easier still if you spend your life delivering babies who do not have a habit of handing you the post as they exit the birth canal. And with many other professions there are undoubtedly also valid mutterings about increased workloads and fewer staff. But there's a difference between not knowing your corporation logo colours and not knowing some really crucial health information that might just save a baby's life, is there not?

The reason it's important, much more important than the 'Red Wine Cures Cancer'/'Red Wine Causes Cancer'-type headlines that newspapers repeat ad nauseam every time someone sneezes is that the UK Office of National Statistics says that formula-fed babies are five times more likely than breastfed babies to develop gastroenteritis, a dangerously nasty stomach infection.

There are mixed views about what whether this is actually linked to formula or other lifestyle factors, but arguably few new mums want to risk putting it to the test.

A key contributor to this sort of infection, it is claimed, is the absolute faff of trying to keep everything sterile all the bloody time. As soon as the powder hits the air, or the bottle comes out of whatever sterilising process you've put it through, it's exposed to bacteria and bam, a nasty dose of the squits (to put it mildly) can become a possibility. In recent years official advice has changed from making up a whole day's worth of formula in the morning to making up each bottle fresh, in order to minimise the amount of time it's hanging around attracting bugs.

Some people think this is bullshit – but nonetheless this change of advice doesn't seem to have been shouted from the rooftops.

'When I interviewed them, many midwifes were unaware that advice now is to make up bottles one at a time – they were telling people you could boil water then cool it in the fridge,' said Dr Battersby.

'It's time consuming – the water has to be the right temperature. Vitamin C, for example, is destroyed by boiling water but it must be over seventy degrees to kill bacteria. But I think in a country like England, where we have good water, and people are educated enough, it's relatively okay.'

Dr Battersby said unequivocally that in her view formula will never be as good as breast milk because there are some tailored ingredients that just can't be mimicked. Formula is high in iron, for example, because supplements are more difficult for babies to absorb than the iron that makes up breast milk.

'But it's not black and white – a mother needs to feed her baby with the method that is best for her, not necessarily the way we agree with.'

She also disagreed with the emotional blackmail that goes with breastfeeding – that you will have a better bond with your child if you do it.

'It annoys me when people say that,' she said. 'What we shouldn't say is "you get better bonding if you breastfeed" – we should say "to have a good bond" do this or this.'

With the exception of mums who cannot feed because of illness such as HIV or surgery such as mastectomy, she also said that many women may be psychologically unable to breastfeed but that this is 'not taken into account'. This can range from those who have suffered abuse, as we talked about earlier, to those who are perhaps under pressure from their partner to do things a certain way.

'Ten to fifteen years ago I had a student midwife with me who was pregnant and her husband had told her he didn't want her to breastfeed,' said Dr Battersby. 'It can be the partner's decision and in some communities they are just not keen.'

Even though for the majority of her academic career she has focused on pro-breastfeeding research, Dr Battersby said she was shunned by some of her peers for carrying out this particular study. Some discredited it because it was funded by a formula company (she claims nobody else would fund it) – and one actually went so far as to tell her she had 'sold her soul to the devil' for even approaching the subject. That doesn't sound too constructive a criticism to me.

'The majority of my research is in breastfeeding but this was something I felt really needed looking into,' she said. 'Some people don't speak to me any more.'

So how about the statistics about formula-fed babies being more prone to diseases such as diabetes later on?

'If you look at how society has altered in the last twenty years, the food we eat and the food we give our babies has altered too. You cannot take one factor and say it's definitely that,' she said.

'We know that the number of young children getting diabetes has increased. Diabetes is an auto-immune disease and exposure to cow's milk (on which most formulas are based) can contribute to the body getting auto-immune failure. There is a reason why they say these diseases have risk – but you need pre-disposition too. You can't say being breastfed will stop you from getting it or being formula fed will give it to you.'

I don't know about you but that made me feel a whole lot better.

CHAPTER 11

Speaking the Unspeakable

You really do take your life in your hands by saying this sort of thing, you know. Because of our situation, we didn't really have a choice in the decision to use formula – I remain convinced that little six-pound Harrison would have ended up in Intensive Care again if we'd carried on listening to the ridiculously generic advice to sit tight and wait for things to fall into place while he wasted away beside me. But even if it had worked out, who knows whether I would have lasted.

Maybe I would have been one of those women who DO make that choice and decide that they just don't want to breastfeed. Is it so terrible that we choose what to do with our own bodies? Cracked and bleeding nipples, mastitis, thrush... just some of the common, agonising conditions that can accompany breastfeeding. And remember, you're doing it several times a day. You can't exactly ask a hungry newborn to be gentle with you. I wonder how many men would put up with all that.

I was going on about it on Twitter one day and got a response from a lady called Inga, a mother of two. 'No one mentioned the excruciating pain,' she recalled of her own experience. She persevered and managed to breastfeed both her children for six months, but her advice now is that the first six weeks are the worst. Six weeks! And let's not forget those are the same six weeks when your newborn baby is ravenously hungry and your exhausted body is desperately trying to heal itself after a pretty major physical event.

My friend Katie lost her husband to cancer very shortly after their second baby was born. She spent a great deal of her time during the week following her little son's birth at the hospice bedside of her partner, who died a few days later. Her mother looked after the baby while Katie was with him.

When the midwife came to visit she asked my by-then-newly-widowed friend whether she was breastfeeding.

'I said that no I wasn't, that I'd just lost my husband and had spent most of my time with him in his last few days,' she recalled.

'The midwife said that was no excuse, and asked me why I hadn't expressed.'

Katie was furious. 'As if I would have sat there in the hospice, saying my goodbyes while attached to a breast pump.'

Woe betide you if you admit that you just don't really want to breastfeed in the first place. I found an entire chat forum on the internet calling for one such woman to be sterilised. I am not making this up.

One of the first times I dared to bottle-feed Harrison in public I was in a coffee shop with a mother and her son at the next table. The little boy, who can't have been more than seven years old, was fascinated by Harrison.

'Look at the baby!' he exclaimed in that stage whisper that only kids think is inaudible to anybody else. 'He's drinking milk! I think I might like baby milk too. Did I have that when I was small?'

'Not out of a bottle you didn't,' hissed his mother, not even attempting the bad stage whisper.

She never made eye contact with me, although I tried my best to eyeball her – not easy when you have both hands full with babies and bottles and you're also trying not to cry. A bitchier person could have found plenty of fault with her, I thought, taking in her WAG tracksuit, abundance of fake bling and general disinterest in her child with the exception of this nasty little exchange. And yet somehow she could leap free range across the moral high ground because (presumably pre-boob job) at some point she'd sat in this very cafe with her baps out.

To be honest, I am still struggling with this.

One night my mum emailed me an article from the BBC News website in which Dr Ellie Lee, founder of the Parental Culture Studies Centre at Kent University, described the official advice regarding feeding methods as 'hierarchical' and called for more honest and open advice about all the ways in which parents can feed their babies.

Shit, I thought, when I read that. *She's hit the nail on the head. I must speak to her.*

It took me all of five seconds to find Dr Lee's email address online and I suspect she may be as addicted to the internet as I am because within about two minutes we'd sorted out a time to chat.

I spent over an hour on the phone to Ellie Lee and came away thinking that either I had just met the world's most convincing conspiracy theorist or there is something a teeny bit Orwellian going on.

The policy underpinning breastfeeding promotion in all countries is a global scheme from UNICEF and the World Health Organization called the Baby Friendly Initiative. Established in 1992 (it arrived in the UK in 1994), its aim is to 'encourage maternity hospitals to implement the Ten Steps to Successful Breastfeeding and to practise in accordance with the International Code of Marketing of Breastmilk Substitutes' according to its website.

Remember that line from the film *Fight Club*, the one that goes 'The first rule of Fight Club is: You do not talk about Fight Club. The second rule of Fight Club is: You do not talk about Fight Club'? The ten steps read a bit like that, but longer. The first step of breastfeeding is: talk about breastfeeding. Second step: TALK ABOUT BREASTFEEDING.

You get the idea.

'The BFI would say it is not out to demonise formula milk. The whole idea is that the biological norm is breastfeeding,' said Dr Lee. 'They think they are fighting a battle on behalf of women over nefarious problematic influence. But I think it's shaped by population politics.'

In her view, extended breastfeeding, especially in developing countries, is a discreet way of implementing something known as 'child spacing' – widening the age gap between siblings – because breastfeeders are less likely to ovulate while they're regularly producing milk. It's all to do with hormones – those released while you're making milk act as a natural inhibitor for those you need to release that all-important egg. UNICEF's official guidelines state that mothers should breastfeed for up to two years (in the UK a minimum of six months is strongly advised, to put it mildly).

See what I mean about sinister? If you look at it that way, women are essentially being told to breastfeed, which conveniently also helps to keep the numbers down. How does that make you feel? If I'd been eating cornflakes at that moment I would have spat them across the room. Fortunately all I had to hand was cold tea.

And yet... maybe it makes sense. Lots of women deliberately use breastfeeding as a form of birth control; it's known as the Lactation Amenorrhea Method, or LAM. The global population is exploding, especially in developing countries, natural resources are stretched – and it's far less brutal than the approach apparently favoured in Uzbekistan, where women are reportedly being sterilised without their consent after giving birth

Still, if this is indeed a covert attempt at population control, Dr Lee rightly said, 'They are never going to put it that way.' And let's be honest, not many new mothers spend those endless night feeds contemplating their role in global politics.

She also pointed to a revival in the popularity of a parenting method dreamed up in the 1950s called attachment parenting. This is the belief that the bond between parents and their children from birth has a huge impact on the psychological development of the child throughout their life. As its name suggests, attachment parenting is all about attachment (no shit, Sherlock) – which includes breastfeeding, co-sleeping, baby-wearing and stay-at-home parenting. I'd never heard of it before my chat with Ellie Lee. And since then, weirdly, it seems to be everywhere – even Alanis Morissette, of all people, was going on about it on a US TV breakfast show recently. And a picture of a mum breastfeeding her six-year-old on the cover of *Time* magazine reignited the debate about extended breastfeeding, a controversial bit of the whole attachment thing.

'Some people diagnose society's ills as a result of attachment failure,' said Dr Lee. 'In extremis some say this failure is also responsible for wars.'

There is no conclusive evidence that any of it is true (in his book *Hitler Among the Germans*, author Rudolph Binion even suggests that, on the contrary, Adolf Hitler was 'excessively breastfed' – make of that what you will). But it also links with a general trend towards a more environmental, less consumerist way of living that has also resulted in ghastly TV programmes in which posh presenters show us how to make our own candles and soap.

Another weapon in the armoury of the pro-breastfeeding brigade is evolutionary psychology, according to Dr Lee.

In a nutshell: 'Human beings are understood as being higher primates,' she explained. 'So we should do things "the way nature intended" as that's what our primate ancestry leads us to do.'

This is also the thinking behind a bonkers diet craze called the paleolithic or 'caveman' diet. It does what it says on the tin. You eat the way people ate millions of years ago and you're healthier, is the theory. My favourite criticism of this approach came from Twitter. 'Cavemen only ate raw food until they learned how to fucking cook' read the tweet (I can't for the life of me remember who wrote it, but if it was you, let me know and I'll buy you a highly evolved beer).

Anyway, back to breastfeeding. The multi-million dollar question: Is breast best?

'Is breast best? I don't think so,' said Dr Lee. 'I think what's best is what people in a particular family think works best. For some mothers it becomes absolutely central to their maternal identity.'

But what about all these terrible health risks, the lower IQs, the ruined stomach linings, the detachment, the overall abject life of misery we're inflicting on our babes in arms?

'It would help if feeding babies was just about feeding babies,' sighed Dr Lee.

'The discourse has departed from anything you would call evidence. A lot of it… it's not made up but it's not far off. Some of the stuff has no basis in reality. The thing about bonding – that is put forward as a baseline argument – that breastfeeding will enable you to bond in a unique way. It's presented as a science but how on earth do they measure that?'

Hmm, that is true. There's no denying that breastfeeding can be a nice moment, when it's not making you feel like you're being stabbed by a thousand red-hot pokers. But so is giving your child a cuddle or letting them sleep on your lap or holding their hands while they try to take their first steps. Does all that count for nothing if you haven't done the boob thing?

After all, if you're a dad, that door is closed from the get-go, right? A new government initiative is deliberately targeting fathers-to-be with the breast-is-best message, said Dr Lee. In the course of her research, she interviewed a lot of formula-feeding mothers.

'The people supporting them in their decision to formula-feed tended to be their own mothers and their husbands – the people I interviewed said they said "you matter as much as the baby". If the husband feels ambivalent and says, "keep trying"... what are you doing to people?'

In Dr Lee's view this is potentially a big threat to family relations at a time when they are needed the most.

I have to say, with hindsight, that if Reece and I hadn't presented a united front over the course of the whole debacle, I could very easily have answered the siren call of postnatal depression, I think.

Truth be told, I am still sad that it didn't properly happen for me. I still don't know why and that in itself drives me mad sometimes. It also forms a hideous dilemma for any future mini-me – I hated the breast pump with a passion, but would it be unfair for me not to put the same amount of effort in, even knowing what I do now? What if it works really well next time? How will I then feel about Harrison?

Whatever happens, I hope I will be much tougher and more decisive around the people supposed to be looking after us. Breastfeeding became an absolute obsession because it was the only thing anyone professional ever talked to me about. I am determined not to teeter on the edge of that dark abyss again over the issue, that's for sure.

If you're reading this because you're in the same place then let me tell you that it will get better, you will get your perspective and your baby will not lose any limbs if you bottle-feed him or her. As the Beatles once said, all you need is love. It's a shame we don't tell each other that more often.

I have two other friends who have babies around the same age as my little boy. Both were breastfed and both suffer with allergies and digestive problems. I am obviously not suggesting this is a result of breastfeeding, but if my son had the misfortune to develop any such thing you can bet your life the formula would have been blamed before I'd even finished saying the word. Bizarrely when I took Harrison to the doctor shortly before his first birthday with a bad cold, I was asked whether he was breastfed. I asked why that was important and didn't really get an answer.

What I now believe very strongly is that the secret of health is all in the genes. With or without the addition of powdered milk.

BIRTH, BOOBS
AND BAD ADVICE

PART 2

Meet some brave ladies who also found themselves to be square pegs in the round hole marked 'breast is best', largely as a result of birth, boobs, bad advice or a combination of the three

BIRTH

Birth issues intervened from the start for these ladies...

Birth, Boobs and Bad Advice

CHARLIE, ALLY AND BABY GEORGE

Charlie suffered serious birth trauma because nobody would listen

While she was pregnant with her first child Charlie simply assumed she would eventually breastfeed despite being 'blissfully clueless' about what it would actually involve. She had an extra reason for wanting to tick all the 'perfect mother' boxes – having lost her own mother at the heartbreakingly tender age of 11 days old, Charlie felt happy that she was finally going to learn first-hand what the word 'mum' was all about.

'I'd spent my whole life really wanting to experience this mystery thing called "mother", and I wanted to be a great mum, the kind of one I'd fantasised about all my life,' she said.

'It never occurred to me I wouldn't breastfeed. I figured it was the most natural thing in the world, so it would be easy. My mother did it; ergo, I would do it.'

Unsurprisingly the holy grail of How to Breastfeed was once again notable by its absence in the run-up to the birth of baby George.

'I don't recall any discussion of breastfeeding in antenatal classes beyond them saying it was ideal for baby to be put on my chest right after birth and breastfeed quickly from there,' Charlie said.

'I hadn't the FOGGIEST what I was getting into. All the info I got was the breast-is-best message; no idea of how to breastfeed or what support would be available (or even the idea it may not work out, which would have prepared me for the fact and saved a lot of shock and guilt).'

With refreshing honesty Charlie describes her first experience of giving birth as 'monumentally shit', and I hope she won't mind me saying that the catalogue of errors which unfolded was so farcical it would almost be hilarious if it wasn't so terrifying.

In late pregnancy she was diagnosed with polyhydramnios, which basically meant George was sharing her womb with a lot of extra fluid. She was told that in her situation the breaking of her waters would be dangerous to the baby and that as soon as it happened she would have to position herself on her hands and knees with her bum in the air.... and then somehow get out her phone and call 999.

It sounds more like a move in an energetic game of Twister than medical advice, and it turned out to be just as useful – but you know how it is. If you were told to wave a chicken in the air and stick a deckchair up your nose, *Spitting Image*-style, you would if you thought it would protect your child.

When the moment arrived, the torrent began and the paramedics were summoned. They soon pointed out they couldn't manoevre Charlie into an ambulance while she was doing a rather loose interpretation of the Downward Dog (for those who know their yoga), and when she got to the hospital the first nurse she saw told her the all-fours routine was all nonsense anyway and then melted away, leaving her and husband Ally bemused and alone.

Despite Charlie's contractions getting more and more painful, as contractions tend to do, the midwives consulted their crystal balls and informed the pair that far from being imminent, the birth was hours if not days away, and they sent Ally home for the night.

'They put me on a ward with three other ladies who were NOT in labour. I spent the next five hours losing my mind as labour intensified. On my own. In a dark ward. With sleeping pregnant women. I ended up sticking pillows over my face to try to quieten the noise I was making during contractions,' Charlie recalled.

When she begged for help she received another pearl of medical wisdom – 'Go to sleep'.

'Go to sleep! Every ten minutes, then seven, then five etc. I was in blinding agony. And all alone,' Charlie said.

Eventually things got so bad that one of her ward roommates (either through pity or lack of sleep) pressed the buzzer again on her behalf. Finally she was checked over and to everybody except Charlie's surprise, she was ten centimetres dilated. The entire box of Dairylea. She was rushed into a delivery room and started to push – but even then she didn't exactly have a captive audience.

'Frankly, after a couple of goes I couldn't see the point. The midwife/doctor who was there to catch the baby kept wandering off mid-push to do something,' she said. 'I kept thinking, *If I push the baby out, he'll fall on the floor!*'

At this point, not only was Charlie in agony and exhausted – she was also absolutely furious.

'I became totally belligerent. I was a bitch (which surprised me; I'm usually quite nice to strangers!). I refused to believe anything they said. I didn't trust them at all,' she recalled.

Fortunately the staff did at least manage to alert her husband – although by the time Ally arrived Charlie was in such a state (she thinks the lack of pain relief had actually driven her mad) that he fainted.

'At one point I begged them to let me die,' she said. 'It took me a long time to forgive myself for saying that – imagine me, having grown up without a mum, wishing that? That's how much I wasn't coping. I hate them for leaving me in that much fear and pain.'

Finally, George made his grand entrance, just in time to avoid the ventouse.

'He came straight onto my chest, and tried to feed in the delivery room, and it didn't work,' Charlie said.

She remained in hospital for two days in order to 'establish breastfeeding' (that old chestnut).

Latching was difficult, positioning was difficult… in a nutshell, 'it really fucking hurt' is Charlie's succinct summary of her breastfeeding masterclasses.

'I'd ring the buzzer for help and the midwife would arrive and shove him on me in a way that I hated (kneading my breasts to get a little colostrum out to tempt him – yergh! Get off me!). As soon as they left, he'd slip off and I could never master getting him latched on.

'Finally, they told me they thought I had overly sensitive nipples and breastfeeding would always be painful,' she said. 'It made a certain sense. I've always hated anything touching them.'

At this stage she realised things had to change.

'I knew emotionally the birth had fucked me up, and now this breastfeeding was making me utterly miserable. I couldn't take any more, and I was sure my emotional state was winding up my baby.'

Charlie decided formula was the only way forward.

'I asked for a bottle. I gave it to George. A massive weight lifted off my shoulders. We went home (though not before one of the midwives told me how disappointing it was that I'd given up).'

Back home, and faced with a wall of conflicting advice and disinterest from her community health support team, it was a family member who eventually talked Charlie through the dark art of formula-feeding.

Charlie was finally able to enjoy her baby and her partner was able to share the pleasure of feeding his little son.

That was until seven months later, when George became dangerously ill. He got an infection between his skull and his brain and in Charlie's words, 'he very nearly died'.

What do you say to a pair of new parents who are somehow finding the strength to watch their seven-month-old baby fight for his life, undergoing gruelling brain surgery and intensive courses of antibiotics?

You might wish them luck, send them love or offer to look after the pet dog/cat/African snail for as long as it takes.

It's not the ideal time to start banging on about breastfeeding, you might assume. Unfortunately not everybody would agree with you there.

'I was asked a lot of questions about his health and development on the neurosurgery ward,' said Charlie.

'A delightful nurse there told me he would have got this mother-of-all-infections because his immune system was compromised by my not breastfeeding him.'

There simply are no words really, are there? It's not like saying you have a hangover because you drank too much wine, or you have a cold because you went out without a coat. Your child nearly died because you didn't breastfeed doesn't really sit comfortably with any definition of the words 'caring' and 'empathy' that I have ever read. Even if it were true – and as we've already seen, there are some pretty strong arguments to indicate that it is not – what was saying it aloud at that moment supposed to achieve?

Not surprisingly Charlie ended up in therapy.

'I could not let go of the emotional side of feeling I'd let George down,' she continued.

'I sat with [my therapist] for an hour a week for a few months and told her, in graphic detail, my experiences in pregnancy, birth and since. She was horrified by much of what I told her, and could see why I was floundering. She helped me a lot. Through her, I realised I had birth trauma. And also that I was not to blame for George's illness. And that it really was okay that I didn't breastfeed beyond Day Two!'

I almost felt like I shouldn't even ask Charlie whether she would attempt to breastfeed any future children.

'I don't know,' she answered candidly. 'I want to say yes, I'll try, even if just for a few days so the baby gets colostrum. I think I will just have to see, give myself permission to be flexible. There's no point bullying myself into it and then not coping at all, and I have doubts as to whether I can breastfeed without it hurting.'

Despite knowing deep down that she would love for it to work out next time, Charlie's determined keep breastfeeding in that part of her head marked *Don't let this ruin your life.*

'My priority is making the best decisions for me to be emotionally at peace, so I can be a good, happy mum to George and the next baby,' she said.

'You're not exactly a great mum when you're crying all the time, cringing when your baby needs a feed and generally wishing you'd never had him.'

JO, DAVE AND BABY ELLIE

Still reeling from a premature birth and feeding issues, Jo then developed a nasty infection herself

Ellie was born six weeks premature and spent her early days in intensive care. Her first feeds were formula, but once her milk came in first-time mum Jo was encouraged to breastfeed her little daughter. Needless to say, with a feeding tube also in her baby's mouth, things did not get off to an easy start.

'I had to do this sort of litmus test to see if the tube was still in Ellie's stomach – which made her scream – and then when I tried to put her on the boob she wouldn't latch,' recalled Jo.

After many attempts to latch Ellie on at every feed, Jo would then be asked to express a bottle.

'At first I had to express into a syringe because there was so little. I remember thinking I'd seen rescued baby hedgehogs fed like that,' she said. (I hated my syringe experience too. I remember bursting with pride when I finally managed to fill an entire one. And then I realised it was only 2.5 millilitres. They don't draw it out of you, by the way, like blood. You squeeze milk into it, drop by slow drop.)

The whole process took 90 minutes and Ellie was feeding every two hours.

'I felt so pressured into it, but I was so keen not to appear like I couldn't cope,' said Jo.

Once the family was back home Jo did manage to switch to exclusive breastfeeding.

'I was really open-minded before hand – all the way through the pregnancy I thought, *I'll try it but I won't beat myself up if I can't do it*. But I went from being open-minded to being obsessed with it – I surprised myself. Our hospital didn't provide bottles or formula (except in intensive care) and all the [other new mums] seemed to be doing it so gracefully.'

However, Jo had one major hang-up – she absolutely dreaded breastfeeding away from home.

'The truth is I could have managed well if I had never left the house. I hated feeding Ellie outside.'

She found herself rushing feeds when she was out and about and she believes that this contributed to a horrendously painful attack of mastitis, a really common infection caused by blocked milk ducts, when Ellie was six weeks old.

'My boob was like a traffic light!' Jo said. 'I was absolutely petrified.'

She was prescribed antibiotics but the pain became unbearable. When she rang her health visitor she was told to continue feeding (the milk flow can flush out the infection). She even begged for a pill to dry up her milk and was refused.

'There is a tablet – I know nothing about it but my mum had it,' she said. (According to the website *Neonatal Formulary*, which provides information about drug use during pregnancy and the first year of life, a drug called bromocriptine was prescribed as a lactation suppressant until 1994 when some pretty scary reports began to surface of users suffering seizures, strokes and heart attacks).

'I couldn't leave the house – I couldn't have anything touching my boob. We had no bottles or steriliser at home and Dave (a policeman) was at work so he couldn't help. He got home at 6 p.m. to find me shivering under a duvet and rang the doctor.'

The doctor told Jo to go to hospital and somehow she managed to drive herself there, leaving baby Ellie at home with new dad Dave. Neither Dave nor Jo expected that she would be admitted, but her infection was so severe she was immediately given a bed and an antibiotic drip.

'I was put on an OAP ward and the baby wasn't allowed in because of tummy bugs going round,' Jo said. 'All the time I was being told to express. I thought, *I've had a premature baby.* I couldn't see why she would want the antibiotics (via the milk). There was nothing wrong with her.'

Jo decided to listen to her gut and did not express from the moment she walked into the hospital. Back home, Dave found himself, quite literally, holding the baby. This meant getting to grips with bottle-feeding pretty damned fast.

'Dave loved feeding Ellie,' said Jo. 'Finally he could get involved in all of Ellie's care. Up to that stage it was just nappies. And she hadn't slept in his arms because they only do that after a feed.'

After two days on the ward Jo's community nurses rallied round and got her home, visiting her every day. After a week on the drip she returned to the hospital to collect yet more antibiotics, but was back down to an oral dose.

There, it turned out that her instinctive worries about the effects of her antibiotic-laced breast milk on Ellie were right all along.

'The doctor said at best she would have got a stomach upset and at worst a very bad one. Yet all the midwives had said to keep feeding,' said Jo.

She and Dave decided not to resume breastfeeding again after the infection was back under control.

'I did it for six weeks and I only stopped because I had horrific mastitis, but nobody – except my mum and Dave – said, "You've done your best." They all looked down their noses and said, "You've stopped." I just needed somebody to say, "It doesn't matter".'

The formula brand they chose was the one they had seen used during Ellie's early days. 'We thought if it's good enough for special care, vulnerable babies... obviously none of the mums there were producing enough milk. The babies were almost all premature.

'I was trying to breastfeed to prove that I could – it wasn't about whether it was best for Ellie.'

Jo was upset that nobody mentioned combination feeding to her.

'I was a first-time mum and I genuinely thought it was all or nothing,' she said. 'I have a friend who bottle-feeds during the day and breastfeeds at night, but it just was not discussed as an option. I would have been able to breastfeed for longer if I'd known it was fine to only do it at home.'

Ellie is now a thriving four-and-a-half-year-old, and for now Jo has decided not to breastfeed future children.

'If I change my mind then it's my decision, but I will tell all the midwives that I'm not going to. I'm sure the health benefits (of breastfeeding) are there, but am I a freak for having a happy, healthy little girl who was bottle-fed?'

Birth, Boobs and Bad Advice

ANNABEL, ROB AND BABY CHARLIE

Lack of support left Annabel feeling a failure for even mentioning the F-word

'I was thinking to myself, *I'll do it for as long as I possibly can. If I like it, maybe I'll be a mum who still has a baby on the boob at eighteen months. If not, then I won't* – but I definitely decided I would try to do twelve weeks,' said Annabel of her decision to breastfeed.

Annabel was already aware that both her own mother and one of her cousins had been unable to do it so she knew that it wouldn't necessarily be easy, but she wasn't alarmed by the prospect – until the breastfeeding 'champion' who ran her antenatal class put the fear of God into her and the eight other mums-to-be in her group.

'It was the worst class we'd ever been to.' She shuddered. 'We all came out shocked by what she was saying. I was angry that she'd made me feel like if I didn't breastfeed, Charlie or I would be losing out.'

The teacher chose not to beat around the bush about how often the group's babies were likely to feed and how long each feed would take, and had some curiously 'hippy' views about the whole thing which Annabel says was far from reassuring.

But one thing she did say to her terrified pupils – to the disgust of one of the husbands present, who is a GP – was that they shouldn't expect to rely on healthcare professionals for support. For Annabel, though, these turned out to be wise words.

'She was trying to make the point that there is help if you want it, but don't expect a decent service from the health professionals. I thought, *that's ridiculous; they are your first point of care...* Really, everything else she was saying was really way-out hippy stuff – she made a lot of women feel uncomfortable about it – but this was the only thing she said that was quite true.'

Unsettled by the teacher, Annabel complained to her community midwife about her. The midwife's reply was strangely revealing.

'Her response was that yes, some people do think she's a bit odd, but they were finding it really difficult to find decent breastfeeding counsellors.'

That is most definitely something worth investigating… but with the birth of baby Charlie pretty imminent by this point, Annabel had more on her mind than why it was seemingly impossible to find reasonable women to run antenatal lessons.

In the event, the birth itself was uncomplicated – Annabel started in the birth pool and ended up having gas and air. Newborn Charlie even did the elusive breastfeeding 'crawl' straight away… but then a serious tear was discovered and the new mum found herself whisked away to theatre in another part of the hospital for a thirty-minute operation that actually took three hours. She was given an epidural and spinal block to cope with the op.

'I was away with the fairies,' said Annabel – wired on endorphins and pain relief. But husband Rob and his new son were left very much in the real world, waiting in the postnatal ward, feeling pretty lost and concerned as half an hour became one hour and then longer.

By the time she returned to her new family it was 8 p.m. and Rob was asked to leave as strict visiting hours meant partners were not allowed to stay. Ninety minutes later a midwife came along to help Annabel get started with a breastfeed.

'Charlie had completely forgotten what he was doing,' said Annabel. 'Every time we put him on the boob he would scream the house down. The midwife was using me as a feeding station, holding his head, pressing it on my boob. I was sitting there prostrate, arms down, wondering whether it was going to work. She kept saying, "I really shouldn't be doing this; you should be doing this yourself," and I thought, *stop using me like a cow, let me have a go…*'

Still, she promised to let her colleagues know that Annabel was having problems and she felt reassured that help was on its way.

And for the first 24 hours, it was.

'During the day there was a nice lady who kept coming and checking and making sure,' Annabel recalled.

The original midwife was on duty again that night and, despite every encouragement, Charlie was still not remotely interested in latching on. So, a formula 'top-up' was introduced.

'Then she finished her shifts and a new set of people came in and I got completely ignored. Nobody even came to ask me whether he'd been feeding okay,' Annabel continued.

However, a visit from a highly acclaimed breastfeeding counsellor was on the cards.

'We'd been reassured by everybody that this hospital was brilliant because it had this great breastfeeding woman,' Annabel said. 'She turned up once for five minutes, but at that point – it might have been Day Two – she said, "Sorry, my shift is ending now. I'll come back tomorrow"... and I never saw her again.'

Annabel had been given a breast pump, but like almost everybody else who's ever hooked themselves up to one, she felt like a one-woman milking machine.

'I thought, *this is ridiculous. I'm spending forty minutes getting a couple of millilitres. I can't pick up Charlie or cuddle him*,' she said. 'I really wanted to be able to bond with him, but how was I going to be able to do that when I'd got a pump stuck to me, and really, he needed more than I was giving him?'

Day Three in hospital and Annabel was still largely left to her own devices.

'I realised Charlie needed to be fed and I didn't know how to do it. It was an awful nightshift. Nobody came to see me.'

Eventually Annabel rang the buzzer and summoned some help.

'I was in tears, saying, "He won't do it. He won't breastfeed. Maybe I need some formula." I was too worried he wasn't getting sustenance from me. They were really reluctant. They said, "Okay, if that's your choice..." There was no reassurance. I felt like a complete failure all the time.'

Charlie ended up with jaundice and Annabel was kept in hospital for even longer while he had blood tests.

'That was the most horrific thing Rob and I have ever had. I was thinking, *that's my fault because I haven't fed him*. Rob was in tears,' said Annabel.

'Night Four was absolutely horrific. I just wanted to go home and be able to take Charlie home. That was when I said, "Look, just give me some formula, please".'

The next day she confided in one of the midwives that she was feeling like a terrible failure.

The midwife said, 'Don't worry, it's your choice. But unfortunately we are a baby-friendly hospital so we have to advocate that breast is best.'

Ah yes, the delightful 'baby-friendly' status, designed to make everybody feel warm and fuzzy, right? At that point, exhausted, frustrated and, let's not forget, pretty poorly herself with a significant post-baby tear, the red mist descended for Annabel.

'I was so angry. I said, "You're telling me I'm not being baby-friendly by giving my baby formula? I can't believe you said that in the same sentence and made me feel twenty times worse." They try to squeeze you into a box, and if you're not in the box, you're not part of the group – they don't treat you as an individual.'

Needless to say, the hospital didn't have much to offer in the way of advice about preparing bottles as the little family finally made their escape.

'They had no leaflets left about bottle-feeding. They kept saying, "We can't really tell you this, we can't really tell you that..." We left feeling quite angry and that we'd been let down.'

New dad Rob was understandably furious at the way his partner had been treated.

'He talked to the midwife when she came round [to the house]. She said, "They let you out too early." But what was the point in me being there if nobody gave me any support in hospital when I'm supposed to be under twenty-four-hour care? I was totally ignored for the last two days.'

Once back home, Annabel's feeding problems continued. Her milk came in but still Charlie didn't latch on properly, and then when he did it he would stop and start so the milk never flowed. Now dealing with 'horrific pain', she decided to go to formula only, but it took five weeks for the engorgement to go.

'You have that lingering feeling that you're completely failing because your boobs are working but something's not connecting with the child,' she said.

And with the move to formula came a different pain – embarrassment about bottle-feeding her boy. Although she says that all eight of the ladies who attended the breastfeeding-class-from-hell with her had problems with it, she was the only one who changed course.

'I felt weird about going to baby groups because I'd be the only one not breastfeeding. I didn't want people to think I thought, *it's going to be a bit gross, so I don't want to do it.*'

Attending baby massage classes, Annabel would leave the room to feed as she was the only new mum with a bottle instead of a boob.

However, little Charlie was doing well – and after a nifty manoeuvre to 'comfort feed' formula to resolve an issue with colic, he began to really thrive and Annabel was finally reassured that he was out of the woods on the feeding front.

'Looking back on the birth, everything went really well,' Annabel now says.

'I felt really good about it. But everything post-birth went downhill quite rapidly. I think that was probably what caused me to be unable to breastfeed. I was so traumatised that things were going quite badly afterwards and I had no support.'

Annabel is unsure whether she would attempt to breastfeed any future children.

'If I try again and it doesn't work, I'm going to go through the same thing: I'll think, *It's definitely me,* and make myself feel low again,' she admitted.

'But if it does work, does that mean I've failed Charlie? I think I'd give my next child exactly the same treatment… but it depends how I feel at the time.'

CASS, JAMIE AND BABY LOLA

Classes, what classes?
Cass opted for a caesarean and was left in the dark about learning to breastfeed

Like so many of the mums in this book, Cass just assumed breastfeeding would come naturally to her. Nobody she knew had ever mentioned any problems, so she thought the whole process must be pretty straightforward.

Cass skipped antenatal classes because she had a planned caesarean birth in store. Nobody mentioned that the breastfeeding class might prove useful, or indeed that there even was such a thing.

Cass's caesarean went perfectly, but when feeding time arrived, she found herself on her own.

'I was left to get on with it. No one helped me at all,' she recalled. 'I tried, by myself, to do it, but Lola wasn't latching on and nothing was coming through, colostrum included.'

It was 48 hours before Lola was weighed. By this point the pair were about to leave hospital but Cass's newly awoken mother's instinct had kicked in big time.

'Lola was hysterical,' she said. 'I knew she'd had nothing, despite the resident paediatrician (a very unhelpful bloke) who kept flippantly telling me, "They can go four days without food."'

Fortunately the midwife who brought the scales took their plight rather more seriously. Cass and Lola stayed an extra night and Cass was introduced to the breast pump. Unfortunately the introduction of a bottle – even with breast milk in it – made Lola even more reluctant to get the hang of actual breastfeeding.

Back at home, hormonal as hell and having a major crisis of confidence,

Cass was happy with the support she received from her local midwives and health visitors.

'They got me to combination feed by encouraging me to use nipple guards. The fact that they were shaped like a bottle helped me get her on, but I never produced enough milk to feed her exclusively by myself,' she said. 'They were very kind and encouraging. That said, it was clear they weren't really allowed to do discuss anything else, such as formula.'

Cass and Lola persevered for ten weeks. By this point the stress and exhaustion were taking their toll on the new mum and she believes the baby was picking up on her bad vibes.

The situation was also affecting her partner.

'He really wanted me to breastfeed and I think felt disappointed by the whole thing,' she said.

'He didn't understand at first how hard it was, but he does now. His obvious stress made the whole thing worse really.'

Cass now believes it's possible her milk was delayed because of the caesarean – but nobody warned her that this might be an outcome of the surgery. Nonetheless, the experience has not put her off trying again in the future.

'If I had another planned c-section, I would just start pumping the minute the baby was born to encourage milk production and I'd do classes beforehand,' she said.

'But if it doesn't work out, I'm not going to be so tough on myself. I know now that it doesn't always "come naturally", though that was never said to me by any healthcare professional, which made the whole experience much more stressful.

'I went through those early days of motherhood feeling like I was failing already.'

BOOBS

Physical issues caused breastfeeding struggles for these ladies – but nobody was prepared to state the obvious and help them move forward

Birth, Boobs and Bad Advice

SHALENE, ANDREW AND BABY ALEX

For first-time mother Shalene a combination of ignored medical history and online peer pressure led to three months of frustration and self-loathing

At the age of 23 and burdened with a batshit insane bra size of 57I, American-born Shalene decided to have breast reduction surgery.

'I knew there was a large risk of nerves and ducts being severed,' she said.

'But when you're twenty-three and a 57I and someone says, "I can cut your breasts off for you," you say, "Yes please, I would like that to happen." ' They removed 1.4 kilograms of breast tissue.

Ten years later, married to a Brit and living in the UK, she fell pregnant with baby Alex and that risk became more real. But after endless research and online discussions with a network called BEFAR (Breastfeeding after Reduction), she was convinced that she would be able to conquer any potential problems.

'A lot of pressure came from myself,' she said.

'I was insisting I could breastfeed. I now know there was a 50 per cent chance that I wouldn't have been able to produce any milk at all.'

At her breastfeeding-focused antenatal classes she mentioned the surgery to a lactation expert who brusquely told her there were 15 ducts in each breast and if a few had been damaged she would be fine.

'I don't know where she got those figures from, but I just didn't question her,' Shalene said. 'You're the size of a house, you're hormonal and scared – you're so vulnerable. It didn't occur to me until months and months later to question it.'

After a five-day labour and a difficult birth, Shalene spent the first night after baby Alex was born in ICU receiving her third pint of blood via a transfusion and having an irregular heartbeat monitored while her 12-hour-old son slept in a glass cot beside her.

'He had the colustrum, but later on Alex started to cry and they said, "Do you want to feed him?" But I couldn't even hold my baby: I had shunts in my hands and feet all pouring liquids into me and I had no energy. So they asked if they could formula-feed him and I was heartbroken – I couldn't even feed my own child.'

The second night, spent tucked up on the maternity ward with four other new mums and husband Andrew at home, Shalene cheerfully described as 'hell on earth'.

'He was screaming and screaming and I just couldn't produce enough milk for him,' she said.

'I was shocked. A voice from the other side of the curtain said, "Why don't you just give him a bottle?" – I didn't care that she'd just given birth; I could have hit her.'

But Shalene padded off to the night shift nurses to ask for some formula, and after just 15 millilitres little Alex was content.

'The next day my husband and I had to ask two midwives how to use bottles because no one had shown us. Even though they had discussed expressing milk in our classes, they hadn't said what to do with the bottles.'

For the next three months Shalene continued to breastfeed her son and top him up with formula, but as he got bigger, the amount of milk he needed also increased and her breast milk volume did not.

He would spend over three hours on the breast and still be hungry. But the breast-is-best message was still coming at her from all angles.

'I would tell every midwife we saw that I'd had a breast reduction and they would say, "Just keep trying." They never said, "It's okay, you can stop." I felt angry and resentful that I had to top up every feed,' she said.

'The minute I had trouble I should have stopped reading online forums – the biggest thing they all said was, "You are doing what's best for your child and feeding them 'crap in a can' would be harming him." That did me in a lot. I hated myself every single time I made a bottle, which was about seven times a day. I would listen to anything – you don't realise that they don't know what they're doing either.'

Shalene hand-expressed and used two different electric pumps. She took fenugreek and brewers yeast, which are said to aid milk production, and even found a recipe for 'lactation cookies' which she ate by the bucketload, much to her husband's disbelief.

'For two or three weeks I didn't wear a shirt – I was constantly either feeding or expressing,' she said. 'And the most I ever got, when Alex was about three months old, was ninety millilitres in one day. At that time he was taking a hundred to a hundred and fifty millilitres per feed. I thought, *if the best I can manage is an appetiser for lunch, where do I go now?* I had defined myself as a mother who mainly breastfed but I realised that I wasn't.'

Fortunately Shalene did have one supportive midwife. 'She said, "Just make sure your kid is fed." I guess when you're dealing with the wider scope of what you can do wrong with a baby, formula doesn't rate that highly.'

A month later the family travelled to America to introduce little Alex to Shalene's family.

'My parents and nieces wanted to spent every second of the day with him and it was incredibly difficult to get the time to pull him away to breastfeed. After a couple of days I realised I didn't mind.

'He's not a maladjusted child – it hasn't broken his heart not getting those three drops per feed from me. I miss that closeness, but he doesn't miss it at all.'

If she and Andrew have another child, Shalene's approach would be to make sure the baby gets colustrum again. She would also commit to 'pumping like a fiend' for a week – but the lactation cookies would probably be off the menu.

'No one ever said, "It's okay to do formula from now on." If that had been expressed to me, I wouldn't have missed out on the first two or three months of my child's life. I was either physically removed from the situation from pumping or I had so much resentment from being stuck on the stupid couch with a kid who would not stop feeding and I couldn't feed him enough.

'In the end, stopping wasn't earth shattering. Alex is obviously very nurtured and well-loved.'

SUE, ANDRE AND BABY DAKOTA-SKYE

Nipple problems caused agony for Sue

'Before I was pregnant the thought of breastfeeding disgusted me,' admitted Sue. 'The thought that my mother had breastfed me... I thought it was animalistic, I didn't fancy it. But as soon as I fell pregnant, I decided I would give it a go.'

Sue felt well-prepared for the challenge of breastfeeding, attending clinics and workshops to find out what support there was.

As soon as her daughter Dakota-Skye was born she was keen to get started – and was delighted when her baby latched on perfectly first time and had a satisfying feed.

Sue's problems began once she was home. Although she thought her milk had already come in, on Day Six she woke up with even more ginormous boobs – and an unusual logistical issue that had arisen as a result.

'My nipples had changed direction,' she said. 'Instead of being straight, they pointed out to the sides.'

By tucking Dakota-Skye under her arm in the so-called 'bowling ball' position, she managed to feed her on the right side, but not the left. Soon she had mastitis in her left breast and the pain was eye-watering.

'The midwife said try anything rather than go on formula, and I didn't want to give up either, but I was in a LOT of pain,' said Sue. 'Dakota was feeding all the time, on for sixty to ninety minutes, off for ten minutes, and then back on. My nipples couldn't take it. I was screaming in pain.

'I remember thinking that I didn't want to give in. I felt it would be a failure to go to formula.'

Sue was concerned that the constant feeding meant she wasn't producing enough milk.

'I was told that you don't run out of milk, that everyone can do it and while it's not a natural process you can learn. It didn't feel natural – I was screaming, she was screaming. As soon as the milk let down I would cry.

'I remember sitting and sobbing. I was in so much pain but thinking, *if you do go on the bottle, you've failed your child, your midwife, your friends.*'

But soon a new feeling swept over Sue – resentment.

'I got angry that she wanted feeding. It got ridiculous.'

At that point she and husband Andre decided that maybe formula wasn't such a bad option after all.

Andre was on his way out the door to buy a carton when their midwife came to visit. She suggested he get nipple shields instead, which he did, but Sue didn't find them helpful. By now – and honestly I am wincing as I write this – half of her left nipple had vanished. Gone! It has never grown back.

In despair, Sue told Andre he would have to go back to the shops and buy formula as originally planned.

'He said, "Oh, I ignored the midwife and got some anyway",' she grinned.

'At first I felt like I'd given up – like when you're training for something, you want to see it through. I loved breastfeeding until it started to hurt. Then there was this huge sense of relief. I didn't rule out going back, but my milk dried up quickly.'

In total Sue had breastfed Dakota-Skye for thirteen days. It didn't help that most of her friends were successful breastfeeders – one even went the extra mile and managed to keep it up until her child reached the age of one.

'The way she talked about it, it's as if she didn't want to put her baby on formula because of the failure,' said Sue. 'Mothers who can do it well must look down on those who can't.'

Sue is currently pregnant with her second child and despite everything she's determined to try again.

'But if I can't do it, I won't think twice,' she said. 'I wish they would be honest and say that some women can't breastfeed very well and you aren't a failure if you don't. You might HAVE to formula-feed, you might not have the option.'

ZOE AND ALEX, MEGAN AND WILLIAM

Zoe was unprepared for the pain of breastfeeding

'It's shocking that it's such a big part of having a baby, and we don't talk about it,' said Zoe on the subject of breastfeeding. 'I've never even talked about this with my mum.

'I remember meeting up with the first mum from our antenatal classes to have a baby and she said about breastfeeding, "God it hurts." I was shocked – I'd never heard that before.'

Zoe and her eldest child Megan set off fairly smoothly on the breastfeeding rollercoaster. They were in hospital for five days to make sure it was all going well and Megan had no problems latching on.

'By the end of the first day it was hurting,' Zoe remembered. 'I thought it was normal. I kept asking the midwife and she helped with positions. I thought it would be fine when we got home.'

Zoe and Megan's homecoming was made all the more blissful by Megan taking a mega-nap as soon as she got into her new surroundings.

'She slept for hours. I thought, *this is okay!*' said Zoe. 'But she was SO hungry when she woke up. I was in agony – it was like hot needles.'

Husband Alex decided to step in and rush out on that familiar panic-buying shopping spree for formula, steriliser etc. – while Zoe called the midwife.

'She said, "You must feed the child." So I did – but every feed was agony. I was crying, bleeding, doubting myself – surely it shouldn't hurt this much?'

Alex was supportive but frustrated. 'He wanted to put her on formula but I wouldn't let him – I was determined to do it,' said Zoe.

After a few difficult weeks she did manage to overcome the pain, feeding mainly on one side – and went on to feed Megan for over a year.

When Zoe fell pregnant with William around a year later she remembered that things had worked out in the end and thought this time things would be better because she knew what to expect. And she was right.

'It was exactly the same again,' she said. 'William went straight to the breast. But I recently found a picture of his first breastfeed and I can see he's in completely the wrong position – and he was put on by the midwife.

'When I was pregnant my boobs were out the door – my boob looked so heavy on William's face. Afterwards I wondered if having smaller boobs would have made it easier.'

She wanted to leave hospital that day – but two weeks later she was back. Things weren't quite the same after all.

'He was tongue-tied but they hadn't picked it up,' she said. 'As soon as they snipped it, it felt different.'

But by then she was also suffering with thrush and mastitis.

'The thrush was a killer for me – every time he fed it felt like glass being shattered all the way up my side. He had it in his mouth and needed medication before each feed.'

'I used to dread the time of the next feed. I could never sit and just cuddle the babies because I didn't want them to smell the milk.'

Unlike some of the ladies in this book, Zoe spoke positively of the support she received at the time. She said she had an 'amazing' breastfeeding counsellor who came to see her every other day and there was lots more information this time around – but after five or six weeks she introduced formula with William.

'I felt guilty for a long time,' she said. 'I did have a stigma about formula. I was quite against it. I don't know if the midwives said it was bad, but it was definitely implied. Is it a maternal thing – a natural urge – the need to breastfeed, or is it what society tells you?'

BAD ADVICE

Sometimes even asking the right questions doesn't get you the right answers...

Birth, Boobs and Bad Advice

ZOE, MARK AND BABY LEXIE

This story was actually written by Zoe herself for the Birth, Boobs and Bad Advice blog but I stopped the proverbial presses to squeeze it in here too because it's just so poignant.

I recently celebrated my daughter's fifth birthday and another big milestone, starting school. As a mum, I never thought I would make it this far – all the excitement and bursting with pride, because it was all so different when Lexie was born.

I have always wanted children. As one of four siblings and as the youngest in a very close knit family I wanted to create that for myself. So when I found out I was pregnant I was so happy. Mark and I had been married for two years (together for ten!) and we felt the time was right. I went through all the obvious things prospective mums do, bought everything and ate everything in sight.

As is usual I was bombarded with 'good advice' and tips from all quarters, especially around the subject of how I was going to feed my new born baby girl. I wanted to breastfeed, but was slightly apprehensive about it. When I spoke to midwives at the hospital, they assured me that it would be the most natural thing in the world and it was be really easy to do. Breast is best and all that.

I started to feel the pressure already.

When Lexie was born by caesarean section on 26 September 2007, the surgeon placed her on my chest and she latched on to my breast like she had always been there. I was elated, exhausted and overwhelmed all at the same time.

Back on the ward, I tried to feed her again, but this time it didn't work. It hurt, it didn't feel right, Lexie was unsettled and crying. The nurses told me I wasn't doing it right, but never attempted to help me.

On the first night, on my own with my daughter, I tried and I tried to get it right, but with a sore wound on my stomach and a chest infection it wasn't working out for me at all.

When I called the nurse and explained that it was painful, again I was told I wasn't doing it right and to stop moaning about it and get on with it. Apparently, I had a hungry baby, and I wasn't producing enough milk. So I asked for a bottle to give her some extra feed. I was met with a grunt and a look of disgust and told to keep on trying until I got it right.

I felt like such a complete failure – on day two of being a new mum. By this time I was so tired and cried quite a lot, why couldn't I do this? Why couldn't I get this right? My nipples were so sore, each feed was like a new brand of torture, the pain was unbelievable. The thought of doing this for six months to a year terrified me.

When I told the midwife about my problems feeding, she called me 'lazy' for asking for a bottle, told me that I had 'given up' and 'taken the easy option'. I was a mess. I couldn't wait to get out of there, as I assured myself it would be fine once I was home.

I was wrong.

At home I carried on breastfeeding with a steely determination but by now I was feeding Lexie all the time just to give her what she needed. It seemed like feeding time never ended, and it was as if I was a cow, albeit a fairly barren cow, but a cow nonetheless!

Lexie by all accounts was a good baby, she slept well, fed well and was really beautiful but I don't remember any of that. My memories of this time are clouded with dark thoughts of my complete failure to provide my daughter with what I was told she needed most – my milk.

Events finally came to a head one day when I tried to express some milk so Mark could feed Lexie. I expressed for an hour and produced nothing but a dribble.

I broke.

I gave up. I sat on my kitchen floor and told my sister I was a terrible mum and it would probably be better for everyone if I died. I had cracked and bleeding nipples, I was exhausted and had nothing to show for hours of feeding and expressing. I wasn't revelling in motherhood, I was spiralling into postnatal depression.

My family went out and bought baby milk and bottles. The guilt I felt was unimaginable. It weighed heavy on my shoulders. I had lasted three weeks of breastfeeding my baby and I couldn't shake off the feeling that I had let her down. Every advert I saw about babies and feeding talked about giving your baby the best start in life with breast milk. Every newspaper article I read talked about how breastfed children did the best at school and had the best immune systems.

Everything got better after I started feeding Lexie with powdered milk in a bottle. This decision changed everything. It seems silly to say it, but everything got brighter, I was happier, I felt human and Lexie was happy as ever.

I'm not the perfect mum, I'm not a natural but I do my best every day and I can't ask for more than that. It's sad to say that the experience I had with breastfeeding and the way I felt about it afterwards has made me decide not to have any more children.

Even five years later, people still ask me if I breastfed Lexie and I get that look when I say I had trouble. I even lie sometimes and say my milk dried up to avoid an awkward situation.

It might seem silly to still feel ashamed about it now but I do. I was out having dinner the other day when a child at the next table started to cry. His mum just picked him up, lifted her top and placed him on her breast, all whilst still eating her food! I looked at her in awe, and five years down the line, the voice in my head still said, *you couldn't do that*.

Looking back now, I'm glad I made the change. It was right for me and my baby. She needed a mum who was with it, able to cuddle her, play with her and bond with her. Not some mess crying in the corner and avoiding her.

If I was to give any advice to a new mum it would be to do exactly what they want to do and feel comfortable doing when feeding their baby.

Mum knows best.

EMILY AND BABY JOEL

Jaundice and bad advice led to Emily's switch to the bottle

'My mum breastfed all four of us. Before I was pregnant I thought it was a bit weird, but that I would do it,' Emily said candidly. 'Then, once I was actually pregnant and started to feel the baby move inside me, I thought I would breastfeed and love it.'

She did buy one set of bottles and a steriliser because it was on a list of preparations she had been given, but didn't give it a second thought.

'When Joel arrived three weeks early, all waxy-skinned and soft, he latched on straight away and I thought, *Yay, I'm a champion mother.* I went home completely elated. I even cooked dinner for my brother and his girlfriend that same night!'

Emily's problems began the next day when she noticed that little Joel's skin was looking slightly yellow. The midwife who came round dismissed her concerns and said the baby was fine.

'He stopped latching on and wanted to sleep all the time,' Emily recalled. 'By the Thursday he slept for seven hours and the midwife shouted at me. She said I had to wake him every two hours to feed.'

By then Emily's milk had come in but Joel was still not playing ball. In the absence of any advice whatsoever she decided to sit tight.

'My boobs got bigger and bigger but he wasn't latching on. I thought the milk would just store up until he needed it.'

Of course what she should have been doing was expressing like mad to keep her supply going – but none of the midwives had bothered to volunteer that information, and at this point she had a more immediate concern: Joel's visibly worsening jaundice.

'When he started to look like the yellow baddie character (Roark Jnr) from *Sin City*, I took him to hospital.'

There he was given blue light therapy. (Yes, really. When I first heard this I thought it sounded bonkers too, but it is in fact a very effective way of curing infant jaundice). But Emily was still told to pick him up every two hours to feed him.

'I also knew he needed to drink lots,' Emily said, having by this point done a hell of a lot of internet research. Drinking helps to flush out broken-down bilirubin, the liver by-product which causes jaundice and is broken down by the light.

'But I had completely empty breasts. He drank what was there but I didn't make any more. I had to convince [the midwives] he needed top-up formula milk.'

It was eventually handed over with great reluctance.

'They were grumpy,' she shrugged.

'They said it wasn't safe to give him a bottle or he would never latch on again. So they gave me a tiny beaker. When I put it to his lips a midwife snatched it away, poured it quickly down his throat and said, "For goodness sake, he can't get used to this."'

After a day in hospital Joel was discharged and Emily spent a further week at home with him, still not really producing any milk. By that point she was frantic and her mother convinced her over the phone to get a second opinion.

'I didn't know whether we were insured or anything but I thought *fuck it* and took him to a private hospital. They looked at me and said, "You are dehydrated, you are exhausted, you need to go to sleep." I hadn't really slept all week. They gave him a bottle and he slept for four hours too, under the blue light.'

When the pair left the hospital the next day Emily had got some rest and her little son no longer looked like a comic book villain.

'He was pink, which was just lovely,' she said.

Unfortunately he wasn't out of the woods yet. After a few days of combination feeding and nappies she cheerfully described as 'explosive', Emily discovered Joel had a milk allergy. So her GP advised her to switch to soya milk formula and remove dairy from her own diet.

'As I was already vegetarian, that hardly made for an easily nutritious diet and I worried constantly about whether my milk was good enough,' she said.

With that problem settled she set about trying to increase her supply again with the dreaded electric pump. She managed to breastfeed Joel exclusively for two weeks but he was 'constantly screaming'.

'I didn't get my milk back but I did get some. One day I had to go to a meeting. I was in London for five hours and I pumped while I was there. I hardly got anything, maybe fifteen millilitres, and I knew then that I didn't produce enough,' she said.

'If I'd known I could have expressed it in the first few days, maybe it would have come in properly.'

By now Emily was angry with the care she had received. She felt that in hospital first-time mums are generally considered to be stupid.

'The midwives were horrible. All they kept saying was, "You will get the hang of it, just breastfeed." I think their attitude was that most mums were just trying to get out of it.

'It affected my relationship with all healthcare professionals for quite a while. I bought my own baby scales because I didn't want to go and get him weighed in a baby clinic. I thought, *I'm not going to be scrutinised and told I'm doing everything wrong.*'

Emily still believes that breast is best but she was also comfortable with her combination feeding, which she continued until Joel was weaned at six months.

'It was never an issue for me. We over-demonise formula. It's like you're giving them dishwater,' she said. 'A bottle is not heroin.'

Joel is now a glossy-haired, pink-skinned, healthy three-year-old and Emily is expecting her second child. This time she hopes for a happier experience.

'If the baby won't eat, I'll express and wait. I'm hoping it will all be fine this time,' she said.

'When I see people tutting about bottles… I saw a celebrity in the paper recently being judged because she was bottle-feeding her baby. I thought, *leave her alone, you've got no idea what's happened to her.* And anyway, it might even have been expressed breast milk!'

Birth, Boobs and Bad Advice

LEAH AND RICK, BABIES OLIVIA AND BEAU

You think feeding one is hard – try feeding two

Leah is a regular contributor to the blog *mumsontheblog.co.uk*. She has written candidly about her life as a mother of twins – and for her, the reality of breastfeeding not one but two babies was not as rose-tinted as she envisaged.

'They made it sound so matter-of-fact,' she said. 'Baby born, plonk on boob, that's it. I thought, *how wonderful*, bought a breastfeeding cushion for two and had visions of just sitting there with a cup of tea and lots of magazines.'

After a relaxed labour and birth – like a true 21st-century mama Leah even managed to keep her Facebook status updated until it was time to push – Leah and her new arrivals Beau and Olivia spent a week in hospital.

'Olivia was so weak, she didn't have the strength to latch on,' recalled Leah. She was also jaundiced and so for the first week she was tube-fed. Her brother Beau, however, seemed ready.

The first time he latched on Leah cheerfully compared with the sensation of having a grater run over her nipples.

'This was not what I had in mind...' she said drily.

Once on, he didn't want to come off. Leah was increasingly concerned about her supply – especially after a sleepless night involving a seven-hour feeding marathon.

'I never felt comfortable and he was always hungry,' she said. 'I had milk but not enough – it wasn't gushing like it should. I always felt I wasn't producing enough. They just told me he wasn't latching on again. I felt awful, like I couldn't do it. I thought I was doing it right and they would say I wasn't.'

At 4 a.m., seven painful hours after little Beau had begun an evening feed, Leah called the nurses in despair. 'One nurse turned round to me and said,

"What are you going to do at home? We won't be there then," ' she wrote on her blog.

The maternity ward was packed and the staff were incredibly busy. During our chat Leah admitted that she often felt like a nuisance.

'It got to the point when they were quite aggressive with him and funny with me,' she recalled.

'I can understand – they were understaffed and very busy. The ward I was on was full, and it's not easy when you have so many people demanding your time. My prenatal care and the birth were brilliant, couldn't have been better. But midwives and nurses are supposed to have a certain empathy and I felt some of them didn't have that.'

She remains grateful to the student nurses who, she says, may have had less experience but showed her more compassion in those dark early days.

Leah, Olivia and Beau were in hospital for eight days and the dreaded breast pump was introduced fairly early on to try to boost her supply.

'They were reluctant to let me formula-feed and to be fair I did want to try [breastfeeding],' she said. 'But I was very relieved to go home. I felt like I couldn't be a proper mother in that environment. It was very hard for me to bond [with the twins].'

Once Olivia had turned a corner health-wise, they were finally free to go. Unfortunately Leah's feeding struggle did not resolve itself once the family was back together at home.

'Someone came round and when she was there it went okay but I couldn't do it,' said Leah. 'I was crying all the time, expressing but getting less and less. I now think the stress wasn't enabling me to produce milk.'

She hadn't really thought seriously about formula. 'I never had a problem with bottles but the main thing they talk about is breastfeeding – that is what you do.'

But after three weeks of anguish, Leah and her partner Rick had an emotional discussion. Leah admitted that she was really concerned that Beau wasn't getting enough food from her and they decided to introduce formula.

'I was relieved when I saw the effect it had on everyone. Beau wasn't crying as much. It wasn't as stressful for me and my boyfriend. I was finally able to get into a routine – and with twins you really need that. Beau had formula every three hours and I could get other stuff done.'

Nearly two years on the twins are healthy and well, Leah and Rick report proudly.

'If we had another one I would try again, but if it wasn't happening I would go to formula,' Leah said. 'When we made the decision, it felt like a massive weight had been lifted from my shoulders.'

SUZANNE

When breastfeeding became a problem for Suzanne, a blog was born

Suzanne Barston runs the blog *www.fearlessformulafeeders.com* from her home in Los Angeles. Because guess what? Things are no different for our friends over the pond.

She launched it in 2009, when her first baby was around six months old. It now gets thousands of hits every month and she has also published a book called *Bottled Up: How the Way We Feed Babies Has Come to Define Motherhood, and Why it Shouldn't*.

'I started blogging because I was thinking about the book, and the more I researched, the more angry I got,' Suzanne said.

Like so many new mums, Suzanne had fully intended to breastfeed her son.

'When he was born, he'd been growth-restricted in the womb, so he came out very thin, and very hungry,' she recalled.

'So it was imperative that we got some nutrition into him. But he was also tired – he'd been stressed out in the womb. When you're exhausted, it's hard to learn a new skill – and latching on is a new skill.'

Only once did Suzanne's baby manage the dark art of latching on.

'The lactation consultants kept saying it was because he was tired, but without sustenance it was hard for him to perk up,' she said.

In addition to the latching on woes, her son was jaundiced – and Suzanne was dealing with that big black dog, Post-Partum Depression, which she says set in within a couple of days of giving birth.

In desperation the family hired a private lactation consultant and had the baby treated for tongue-tie, but nothing helped with the tricky issue of latch-on.

'I exclusively pumped for about a month,' she said. 'And he was so sick. He cried all the time, he had diarrhoea, when you gave him a bottle he would drink for a bit then pull away and scream, then drink a bit more and scream again.'

Eventually he was diagnosed with a milk protein allergy. So Suzanne decided to eliminate dairy from her diet altogether but it didn't seem to help.

'A specialist suggested we try hypo-allergic formula for twenty-four hours,' she said. 'Within four or five hours he was a different baby. I have since learned that this is very typical with severe milk protein allergy: the second you take away the catalyst their bodies can clear it out very quickly.'

Dealing with her own psychological feelings of failure, Suzanne began to look more closely at the breastfeeding versus formula debate.

'People have lost all compassion over it,' she argued. 'I hate to get hysterical about it but I think things have got progressively worse. There is scary chatter around such as making formula prescription only – and worse. Even if you believe it makes that much difference (and I personally do not), that does not mean you can take away the choice for women.'

Like so many of the women in this book, Suzanne is angry about the lack of information available to formula-feeders.

'There is such a bias in getting information,' she said. 'You can get it from the formula companies, but they're not doctors, they are providing a commercial product.'

The rumour mill abounds – like me she has been unable to pinpoint the source of the mythical 4 per cent (bizarrely in the USA it is said to be between 1 to 3 per cent) of women who are said to be physically unable to breastfeed. Suzanne thinks it has something to do with one single study once of women in Sweden. Perhaps we will never know.

She also feared for her son's health as he was missing out on all those precious antibodies we are always told other mums are pumping out.

'I was convinced we shouldn't take our son out for the first six months because he was immuno-compromised from formula-feed,' she said. 'But it turned out he was never sick for the first three years of his life.'

Suzanne recalls a tragic story from December 2011 about a formula-fed baby called Avery Cornett in Missouri who fatally contracted Cronobacter sakazakii – a very nasty bug that causes chronic infection. There was a national outcry, the formula brand was pulled off the shelves... and then it transpired that the bug had been introduced after the formula left the can. At the time CBS news reported that the US Food and Drug Administration sees four to six cases a year of this horrible illness – dreadful, but hardly an epidemic.

'There are rare breastfeeding-related deaths too – you occasionally hear about babies being smothered by the mother's breast, for example,' said Suzanne (a quick search online reveals numerous examples of this – perhaps most notably the sad case of a four-week-old baby who died while breastfeeding on a flight from Washington to Kuwait). 'But there isn't the same sense of panic as when formula-feeding is involved.'

Here in the UK, Dr Ellie Lee (remember her?) sat in on a meeting of the Food Standards Agency where they explained their decision to change the official advice for preparing formula milk bottles from making them up in advance to only making them up just before use. The FSA's rationale was based on minimising the risk of introducing this nasty sakazakii bug to infants – which sounds like a noble enough cause.

However.... 'The number of incidents possibly related to this bacteria, globally, ever, is less than a hundred,' said Dr Lee.

'It is an utterly risk-averse claim that since formula milk isn't sterile it must constitute some level of risk... even though there is no sign it came from the milk.'

Thus the current advice that bottles of prepared formula milk be discarded for hygiene reasons 'has no basis in any study, ever' according to Dr Lee.

'I remember thinking the only winner is the formula manufacturers who sell those expensive ready-made cartons,' she said.

Ka-ching.

Over in the US, meanwhile, Suzanne was astonished when she wrote a blog post about colic and in a reply someone innocently suggested that breastfed babies never got it.

Even *my* most prolific breastfeeding friends laughed long and hard over that one.

Birth, Boobs and Bad Advice

MILK MAKERS

These next three stories have a different ending.
The following ladies were also determined to breastfeed and they did get there in the end.

But I think they also have a place here because these women also found themselves faced with ridiculous scenarios. So far we've bitched about breastfeeding bullies. Well, they left Gill, Louisa and Kirsty utterly alone – despite their cries for help.

GILL, IAN AND BABY LILY

Geography left Gill slipping through the net

'I basically gave it zero thought, I was so naïve,' says Gill now. 'I just thought yes, I'd like to [breastfeed]. I'll do it.

'I have no complaints about my antenatal appointments, but breastfeeding was only mentioned once. They asked if I wanted to and I said yes – and that was it. I think they should have said, "You might need a bit of help".'

(This reminds me of yet another mad moment in my own antenatal classes when we all had to waddle into position along a line depending on how hard we thought breastfeeding was going to be. The lower end, down by the changing mats, was 'hard' and the upper end, up by the nice toys, was 'easy'. We almost all stood innocently either in the middle or in the 'easy' bit at the top. I remember talking to my husband about what on earth could possibly be so difficult about it. Nobody enlightened us.)

Gill only fed baby Lily once in hospital (after a 'great' birth – Gill's secret weapon was hypnobirthing techniques) because little Lily spent most of her stay at Hotel Maternity Ward fast asleep.

'A midwife came in, saw me feeding and said, "Great." I thought, *obviously that's it. The baby just pops on.* They said nothing about making sure the baby latches on that way or anything.'

The problems started a couple of days later, at home, when Lily's latching technique started to take its toll.

'I was in the worst pain I have ever known – and I'd just given birth without any pain relief,' said Gill. 'After two days she was coming towards me and I knew how much it would hurt and I felt like pushing her away. I thought, *I don't want you on me because it hurts so much.*'

Gill decided to grit her teeth and wait for the imminent arrival of her health visitor – who was surely due any moment now, right?

Wrong – thanks to a time-honoured admin cock-up nobody came. When Gill eventually rang the service her name wasn't even on the register, she thinks perhaps because she lived in one region but gave birth in another.

It was three days before the health visitor decided to do the decent thing and pay a visit.

'By this stage I was in agony. Lily was losing weight as babies do but she also had jaundice, and the way to deal with that is you have to feed every two hours,' Gill recalled.

'Feeding every two hours is completely exhausting – the feed takes an hour. You've got no time, you get no sleep, plus the pain in your nipples... they were cut and cracked.'

The health visitor promised to send a breastfeeding expert but, *quelle surprise,* yet again nobody turned up.

By this point it was nearly Christmas and there was snow on the ground. In desperation, Gill and Lily trudged round to their local SureStart Centre breastfeeding group.

'At first I just saw a room full of women breastfeeding their children,' she remembered. 'I burst into tears and thought, *how am I ever going to do that?*'

Fortunately, the women were able to help Gill, both practically and emotionally.

'It was the first flicker I'd had that others found it hard too,' she said. 'This woman said, "Don't worry, we've seen this loads of times," and showed me loads of positions.'

However, with Christmas looming large, the centre shut for the holiday and Gill and Lily found themselves without any help again (Seriously? Where were they all? Maybe you have to play hard to get).

'Christmas was my lowest point,' she said. 'I felt like I was really failing in every way. I thought, *this is what I'm supposed to be good at as a mum. I'm a total failure.* I'd done well at work, I have the kind of job where I'm making decisions all the time, and suddenly I just didn't know what I was doing.'

Now she was also worried about her supply, so she gave Lily formula top-ups with a syringe, which she found 'horribly depressing'. While Gill didn't mind the formula itself (hey, she's another child of the '70s, we were all on it) she hated the syringe, which she was using to avoid this crazy 'nipple confusion' thing that I remain really unconvinced by.

'I thought, *my baby isn't a little waif wandering off the street*,' she said. 'It seemed wrong. But I didn't feel bad about the formula itself. I think it's demonised. I didn't feel there was anything wrong with that.'

Gill continued the battle to breastfeed – but the turning point came when her husband Ian burst into tears.

'It was shocking. He's this macho rugby playing fellow... and he just said, "I don't know how to help." '

Some hasty Googling produced a local lactation consultant who did what the health visitor should have done in the first place and came straight round.

'The main thing she said is, "You don't have to do this, your baby will still be fine",' said Gill.

(That was the last thing I expected to hear a lactation consultant say – well done, that woman.)

'I had a good talk with her, how I felt it wasn't natural, it felt absurd to keep doing it when it hurt so much.'

Amazingly the consultant agreed with her. But she also taught Gill and Ian some pain management techniques and Gill found that the pain did ease and she was eventually able to breastfeed without the top-ups.

'If we have another child, I would try it again,' said Gill. 'With the knowledge I have gathered it wouldn't be such an uphill struggle.'

Not surprisingly she feels that very little of her care was actually aimed at her as a parent.

'I love my daughter more than life itself, but (the care) feels like the cult of the baby – what about the mums?'

Birth, Boobs and Bad Advice

KIRSTY AND D'ARCY

Kirsty was a slave to the breast pump

Kirsty felt she had missed out on breastfeeding first time round, as her older daughter Caitlin was born prematurely and her milk didn't ever come in.

'She was in hospital for eight weeks and I was pumping, but I could see in the fridge that everyone was getting about twenty millilitres and I would only get two,' she recalled.

'I felt like I never had a choice with the eldest. So this time around I was worried. I said I would try for a week and if I could do it, great; if not, I'd use bottles.'

Despite a long labour which ended in an emergency caesarean, little D'Arcy latched on straight away, and after treatment for tongue-tie, the pair were sent home. However, just like me, Kirsty never experienced the gigantaboob moment.

'I would feed her but I knew something wasn't right,' said Kirsty. 'She would feed for hours and I would squeeze my breasts and nothing would come out. Everyone said you don't run out [of milk] but my boobs were empty – I *know* you can.'

As time went on, health visitors expressed concerns about D'Arcy's slow weight gain, but as Kirsty had decided to press on with breastfeeding, her GP referred her to the local Bosom Buddies group for support.

She did not find it to be the haven she was hoping for.

'If I'd been twenty-one years old I would have been so intimidated,' she said. 'It was cliquey, there were lots of older kids and toddlers, and nobody was talking about breastfeeding.'

However, two positive things did emerge from the excursion. The group leader noticed that D'Arcy's tongue-tie hadn't been fixed properly, and she loaned Kirsty a breast pump to try to stimulate more milk production.

Determined, Kirsty spent the next ten weeks hitting the pump big time – getting her own on eBay after a sudden call came from Bosom Buddies, demanding their loaned pump back straight away.

'I don't know how I got the inclination to do that. I would get three ounces a day, and it became an achievement to beat that. Eventually I got ten ounces – but I would pump every hour once D'Arcy went to bed.'

Kirsty's obsession took over the whole family.

'My other daughter got upset. She would say, "You're pumping again, Mum – you haven't just got one daughter, you have two."'

She was also feasting on fenugreek like it was going out of fashion, munching twelve tablets a day as it is said to help breastfeeding women produce more milk. The recommended dose is one pill with each meal.

'I don't know whether it worked but it got to the stage where I was too scared to stop taking it,' admitted Kirsty.

Somehow she made it to six months although D'Arcy weaned early.

'I don't know how I did it,' says Kirsty now. 'I feel proud – but if I had another and I had to pump, I wouldn't. I don't like people who drum it into you that you should breastfeed. Every baby is different.

'I know a boy who's been poorly and his mum has been told it's because he was bottle-fed. I've now done both and I can't say that Caitlin has not benefited [from not being breastfed].'

Let down by the professionals, Kirsty says she found the admiration and encouragement she needed from peers on the internet.

'My biggest support has been Twitter,' she said. 'I feel sorry for first-time mums – especially those who aren't confident enough to speak up.'

LOUISA AND OLIVER

A combination of conflicting information and yet another case of mastitis shook Louisa's desire to breastfeed her first child, Oliver, now five

Louisa admits that the pressure to breastfeed came mainly from within. 'Everyone has their own preferences and ideals,' she said. 'People feel very strongly about what they think is right around parenting.'

But things took a turn for the unexpected when Oliver ended up being born by emergency caesarean. When it came to feeding, he had difficulty latching on from the get-go, while the pair were still in hospital. Louisa found that not all the staff were that desperate to help.

'There were a couple of nurses who could get him on, and one breastfeeding counsellor, but she was only there every other day,' she remembered. 'I asked a care assistant for help and she said, "It's not my job." I said, "Whose job is it?" and she said, "The nurse, but she's on her break." '

A month after leaving hospital Louisa was hospitalised on Christmas Eve with a bad case of mastitis – and this turned into a proper circus. Her treatment involved an operation, the wound was fitted with a drain, and when she was discharged, on a Sunday evening, she was told to get the dressings changed daily at her GP practice. Come Monday morning, she found the GP had other ideas and said there were no appointments. When she insisted, the first nurse to see her told her the operation had gone wrong and would have to be re-done. The hospital disagreed and an argument erupted between the two.

While all this was going on, Louisa tried to continue breastfeeding but could only manage it from the uninfected side. She supplemented Oliver's food with formula.

'I felt an enormous amount of shame about the mastitis,' she said. 'After having the emergency caesarean I felt like I couldn't even give birth, the baby was literally cut out, so I felt I had to be able to breastfeed to fit the earth mother ideal that I wanted motherhood to be. Instead I'd had an infection. I felt contaminated, bad.'

After the operation Louisa could only express, but using an electric pump was 'like a nail going through my nipple', she winced. With not much milk being produced, she eventually abandoned the process.

Like Kirsty, Louisa felt a lack of support from the postnatal team throughout.

'I felt as though there wasn't much interest either way – the health visitor was only interested in filling in the chart,' she said. 'They weren't there for me.

'The obsession with weight and writing in the book takes away from what mothers need – reassurance, help, affirmation.'

When she fell pregnant with her daughter five years later, Louisa was very wary of the conventional support network.

'I was really emphatic that I went to a different hospital. It felt like the only way I could take control,' she said. ' I was surprised when the community midwife was good, but part of me was still reticent about engaging with the health centre.'

This time around she was also happier with the baby clinic, which is now held in her local Children's Centre rather than at the GP surgery with its queues of mothers waiting in line all able to hear each other's consultations.

'But I do feel like I'm going there to be judged about whether the baby has put on weight,' she admitted. 'It seems to be their only concern. I'm more concerned about whether she is happy. I've only been asked once whether she smiles.'

Louisa is happy that she has been able to breastfeed – although even without any problems second time around her milk took two weeks to really come in.

'It feels like a nice way to spend time with my baby,' she said. 'I do still think ideally breast milk is best, but it's not always possible.'

EMILY, KEVIN, WOODY AND MAYA

Permanent pumping got Emily through breastfeeding difficulties

'I was determined to give it a go,' said Emily of her decision to breastfeed her first child. 'I was told it was best; I believed it. But I didn't research it, which is quite unlike me – I was quite chilled out about it.'

Emily recalled coming away from an antenatal talk on the subject thinking that it might be difficult for a few days. Then, when one of the first of her antenatal buddies had her baby, she was surprised to find her mate was reluctant to breastfeed in public.

'I thought she must be embarrassed,' says Emily now. 'I didn't realise it was because it hurt. Then I saw another friend feeding with tears rolling down her cheeks – I still thought, bolshily, that I would be okay.'

Emily's son Woody was eventually born on a Sunday morning, and by Monday he was jaundiced, after spending his entire first day in the outside world fast asleep.

'If they don't feed, they get jaundice – but we couldn't wake him to feed him,' she said.

'That first night they said, "We have to get some liquid into baby," grabbed a formula bottle and rammed it into his mouth. My boobs were killing me. I expressed some colostrum – not even a teaspoon – and we fed him that by syringe.'

News of the formula incident did not go down particularly well with the day shift.

'Next morning, a midwife came in and hit the roof,' Emily said. 'She said, "We are trying to establish breastfeeding!" But Woody wasn't bothering to latch on really, he was nibbling, which I think was why it hurt so much.'

Two days later the pair were released from hospital – but Woody had still only had that one bottle of formula milk. So Emily chose to be transferred to a different hospital, where her newborn was introduced to the sippy cup.

'What a joke that was,' said Emily drily. 'I kept attempting to breastfeed but it was very, very painful. My milk hadn't really come in. When he was a week old we left the hospital. I felt like I was breastfeeding but I was still in agony.'

Organised Emily had actually managed to buy a bottle steriliser before Woody was born, in case of just such an emergency.

'I'd put it in the shed. I decided I would have to go and get it – but I'd told my husband not to let me do it the first time I asked.

'I kept saying to myself, "If I can just get through this pain that everyone else has gone through, it will be okay. It's like giving up smoking, or not phoning an ex".'

Emily was reassured by her peers telling her it hurt them too – but still struggling to handle the pain, which was particularly excruciating on her left side.

'I couldn't bear to feed outside because it hurt so much. I would cry, I hated it. By the time Woody was six or seven weeks old I was pumping the left side and not using it to feed at all. But when you pump you have to pump more regularly to keep it going.'

Part of the pressure Emily felt under was that the new family had booked their first holiday *a trois* – to Majorca.

'I was determined to keep going because I didn't want to use the water there. The day we came back was such a relief.'

Emily had enough breast milk stored from her pumpathon to use for another month – but her New Year's resolution that year was not to get hung up on breastfeeding if she ever fell pregnant again.

Despite this, Emily spent the last two months of her second pregnancy using a nipplette every night to 'correct' one of her nipples, which was flatter than the other (this cunning contraption apparently 'sucks' inverted nipples back out again... yup, I'm wincing yet again, are you?).

And at first her hard work seemed to pay off – when the time came, daughter Maya latched on straight away.

'I was delirious that she'd done it,' Emily said. 'It was a big achievement. This time I was regimented about it – as soon as she woke up, we would try to feed. I was determined to make it happen.'

Two days later, however, the pain was back. After leaving hospital, Emily's first outing with her new daughter was to a Bosom Buddies group.

'I was so desperate to get there in time for her feed, someone reversed into me on the way there and I just kept driving,' she said.

But they had no answers. 'The people there were lovely… they watched me and said that it shouldn't be hurting this much.'

After three weeks, Emily was getting desperate. She had grown to dread feeding time and was worried that it was affecting her bond with her hungry little newborn.

So she decided to go down the same route as Kirsty, abandoning breastfeeding altogether and instead becoming a full-time pumper – although researching the idea proved fruitless.

'I couldn't find any advice on 100 per cent pumping. The breastfeeding counsellor pooh-poohed it – said my body would not keep up,' she said.

'I only went to friends' houses where I could pump,' Emily recalled. 'Forty minutes each side, all through the night. By four weeks I was in a rhythm and at six weeks I considered going on. I loved feeding her with milk from the bottle – I really bonded, I could see her – and suddenly I liked her, I saw her enjoying her food.'

Like Kirsty, though, there was a problem – the continuous pumping was affecting Emily's other child.

'The effect on Woody [by then] was enough – I was really tired. I think you can do 100 per cent pumping without another child. I never got dressed.'

With the support of her own mum and husband Kevin, Emily gave up.

'There was a sense of loss. But I feel hand on heart that I did everything I could – and I'm glad I did. I still felt jealous that breastfeeding had worked for other people and not for me.'

Like Sue, Emily bears a distinctive physical reminder of her fight to feed.

'After I finished feeding Maya my nipple went in completely – and it's never come back out. They said it might have been caused by trauma.'

AND FINALLY...

A word from the wise

My own son is now a happy, healthy toddler who eats pretty much everything, especially my hairbrush. I find myself reading back those early chapters about our struggles astonished that I actually wrote them myself.

But I still get the occasional reminder that there are lots of people out there who will have no qualms about telling me I did completely the wrong thing. A friend of a friend on Facebook told me the other day that anyone who speaks out in favour of formula is merely 'justifying their inferior choice' – but it's okay, she's not a judgemental person: she went on to say.

'Thank goodness for that', I replied - but I'm not sure she got the irony.

Someone else who knows all too well about this unashamed bottle-bashing is Dr Joan Wolf, a renowned American academic and feminist who wrote a book called *Is Breast Best?* in which she argued that it wasn't. As you can imagine, she may as well have organised a house party with an open invitation to internet trolls – and this was in the early 2000s before everybody with a smartphone could get online and launch a global war of words from the comfort of the number 27 bus.

Dr Wolf and I spoke on Skype – she in her book-lined US university study and me in my baby's nursery, with, I discovered afterwards, a bit of baby sick on my left shoulder. Neat.

Dr Wolf calmly described the public response to her book as 'overwhelmingly negative... really quite hostile on the blogosphere' (I suspect that was a bit of an understatement), although she said she received many private letters that were positive.

'There is a large population of women out there who believe the discourse has become insane,' she said. (Have you noticed that only academics can use words like 'discourse' and still sound cool?)

In her book Dr Wolf approached the breastfeeding/formula debate with the intellectual equivalent of a rather large, rather swingy wrecking ball.

'It seems okay to say breast is best, but if you want to formula-feed, don't worry about it,' she told me. 'So when I make the claim that the evidence for that is flimsy... well, that is problematic. I have broken a rule.'

That's putting it mildly. I felt like I'd just used the C-word in front of my parents and I was just writing down what she said. But I was also already a little bit in love with Dr Wolf.

'I started researching the book in 2004/5. I started reading the science... There is no evidence that breastfeeding itself makes a difference,' she said, just like that, like you might say, 'The sky is blue' or 'Pass the salt'. No ifs, no buts.

So I'll add the 'but' – even though I have questioned that myself, it is still one hell of a claim to make, given the fuss everybody's made over breastfeeding being 'best'.

She backed down... a little. Okay, breastfed children do tend to be 'slightly' healthier, she conceded.

'But is that the breastfeeding itself?' she argued.

'We don't have the evidence that it is. My claim is: if you have parents who wash their hands, who don't take their child to the supermarket at five p.m. when it's packed with people coming from work... perhaps women who choose to breastfeed demonstrate these behaviours.'

She's right, when you think about it – it's pretty difficult to pin down one lifestyle factor in most situations unless the evidence really is overwhelming, and, as you'll see in a minute, it doesn't appear to be here. But even still, this does open up the rather strange notion, occasionally bandied around in the newspapers, that there's a class divide, or perhaps simply an intelligence divide, between breast- and bottle-feeding parents. I'm still not convinced that it exists – if we go down that road do we also then say that bottle-feeding mums have lower pain thresholds or different shaped nipples? Hmm – now there's a research project for somebody brave.

Here's an example of the evidence she cited: you probably don't need me to tell you that breastfeeding is widely believed to 'protect' infants from what doctors call Gastrointestinal Infections, or GI (or what my family calls a nasty dose of the squits). A study published in the Journal of the American Medical Association in 2001 carried out in Belarus (a city that for some reason crops up quite a lot in this sort of thing. Who knew?) certainly seems to support this.

On the face of it, the statistics are alarming. Forty per cent more breastfed babies in that study got a GI. Gulp. Forty per cent!

But before you throw away the steriliser, argued Dr Wolf, look at the actual figures behind the headline.

'Thirteen per cent of babies who were not breastfed had one or more GI infection. Nine per cent of breastfed babies had one or more. Yes, it's a forty per cent difference, which you think is massive, but actually you are talking about four diarrhoea infections per one hundred babies. That means you need twenty-five babies to be breastfed in order to prevent ONE diarrhoea infection,' she claimed.

As odds go, in a country with clean drinking water (that bit is absolutely crucial) those numbers aren't exactly overwhelmingly worrying. Frankly I don't know a single one-year-old here in the UK who hasn't had diarrhoea, whatever the hell they've been eating (actually that in itself can cause the problem. You can sterilise bottles until the end of time but you won't stop your little beloved eating the mouldy Cheerio he or she found down the back of the sofa while your back was turned). Yes, I do realise that it is potentially a great deal more serious for small people, and just to reiterate, this is very much dependent on the state of your national water supply. But in the grand scheme of things, here in the UK it worries me less than, say, a red-rash-that-doesn't-fade-under-a-glass would.

Dr Wolf also shot down the theory that breast milk is a superhero in liquid form, fighting germs wherever it finds them.

'We know there are antibodies in milk, we know they line the baby's gut and can fight bacteria. But we don't have evidence that they go anywhere else in the body. Are they ultimately excreted along with everything else?'

Personally I'd rather not get too close to the contents of a newborn nappy – even now, and I've been sprayed with the stuff – but it is an interesting point.

At the start of this book I wrote about 'the science bit' and said flippantly that I was unable to find it. At the time I was surviving on hormones and no more than two hours' sleep at a time. To be honest, the science bit could have been written in six-foot letters on the side of my house at that point and the chances are I might have missed it. But Dr Wolf couldn't find it either, which did wonders for my confidence in my own rather compromised investigative journey at that time.

So why has breastfeeding become such a proverbial hot potato?

'The expectations of motherhood in the twenty-first century are unlike anything we have had before,' she argued.

'So much of the breastfeeding battle is about women demonstrating that they are wonderful mothers. Mothers are other mothers' fiercest critics... we believe we can create the perfect environment for us and our children... and there's a belief that if we get sick, it's our fault.'

That certainly struck a chord. If my son so much as sneezes I find myself running through a mental checklist of what could have caused it. 'Because sometimes our bodies just do weird shit' isn't on that list, but it really, really ought to be.

'There is no evil ingredient in formula,' said Dr Wolf (I would love to see the look on the face of the doctor who raised his eyebrows when I presented my son with his first cold and he asked me whether he had been breastfed).

Its manufacturers are certainly no angels, however, and the way in which milk has been aggressively marketed overseas is a source of much anger.

'I'm not out to line the pockets of the formula industry – formula is produced for profit by an industry that has behaved very badly in the past,' said Dr Wolf. 'But that industry itself says that breast is best, which is remarkable, given the very weak associated evidence. It's like Nike saying, shoes are bad, but if you have to wear shoes, wear ours.'

Ultimately Dr Wolf would like to see some perspective brought back into the debate over infants and their diet.

'I would advise women and their partners to understand that how you feed your baby is one choice among millions you are going to make,' she said. 'The choice is not nearly as loaded as you think it is – and in the scheme of things, whether you choose to breastfeed doesn't make that much difference at all.'

So. Go and have a cup of tea, and a biscuit – two or three or the whole damned packet if it's one of those days, and, most importantly of all, don't worry. You're not the first or the last and everything is going to be all right.

CALLING THE MIDWIFE

The Royal College of Midwives has its say.

I very nearly didn't write this bit of the book. I put it off and tried to convince myself that we didn't really need it. Perhaps, deep down, the last thing I wanted to do, selfishly, was put myself in the path of yet another midwife. But the irritatingly thorough journalist in me kept nagging away that really, after all this dissatisfaction and in some cases (yes, okay, mine), midwife bashing, it was only fair to let the official folk have their say.

To be honest, even once I'd made that decision it nearly didn't happen. It took several weeks of badgering the poor press office at the Royal College of Midwives (RCM). Eventually they put me in touch with a lady called Janet Fyle who is Senior Policy Advisor at the RCM. Except somehow the message hadn't quite got through to her about what I wanted to discuss, and when we finally did speak, initially she wasn't particularly happy about this bolshy woman phoning her up to bend her ear over breastfeeding policy.

All the signs suggested that we were not going to get on. However – and I think to the surprise of us both – we did. I spent over two hours talking to Ms Fyle and we even swapped phone numbers at the end of it. We might actually become friends (until she's read this book, at least).

I started by asking her why so many women feel unhappy about the support they receive with breastfeeding.

'It's a difficult one, to be honest with you,' she said. 'The research comes up time and time again that one of the reasons women give up breastfeeding is because they don't have continuous support.'

Because women spend less time in hospital than ever after having their babies, and there are fewer community midwives employed by budget-conscious Primary Care Trusts than there were in less austere times, that support is diluted, she said.

'I'm not giving any excuses that shortage of staff is the main factor, but it is one factor, from my perspective. Although it should not be a reason for women not getting support.'

'But I have met women who have been absolutely desperate to stop breastfeeding,' I said. 'All they want is for someone to tell them it's okay to stop trying. Why doesn't that happen?'

'The midwife doesn't want to tell the woman to bottle-feed because it is not her place to do so,' said Janet.

'Maybe the woman is thinking, "I want the midwife to say to me, 'Just bottle-feed.' " But I wouldn't think in the midst of that woman trying to get support and wanting to try [to breastfeed], somebody should undermine her confidence by saying, "Give up." '

There's a logic there I suppose – but the issue for me is still that breastfeeding is considered the norm until you, the knackered, hormonal, emotional and scared new mum, somehow finds the strength to challenge the status quo and decide that it isn't working out for you. I don't know many first-time mothers with newborns who have historically started revolutions. It took me over a year just to write a sodding book about the subject.

'The key issue around formula-feeding is about the woman making the decision independent from anybody else. If the woman comes to the midwife and says, "I have thought about this and read about it and this is what I want to do" – the midwife needs to respect that decision.

'We are not supposed to be pressuring women,' Janet added.

I can't help but think that this is a slightly idealistic scenario. Unsurprisingly Janet, like most midwives, firmly believes that breast is best. While she says that midwives need to respect the decision of the mother regardless of their personal views, I imagine that in reality that's not so easy after a long shift on the labour wards. Even in my line of work, screaming "Are you out of your fucking mind?" at someone you fundamentally disagree with is sometimes difficult to resist. And I haven't spent ten hours coaxing a life form out of their insides first.

Anyway, whether she personally believed the entire breast-is-best rhetoric or not, Janet spared me the chat about breastfed babies and immortality.

Interestingly the only issue she brought up as a potential hazard regarding formula-feeding was the bacteria issue.

Not everybody thinks there's a strong case for that either, I said, thinking of Dr Ellie Lee and Dr Joan Wolf.

'It is fine for anybody to dispute the evidence, but the most important thing is not about whether they dispute the evidence or not, it's that mothers know they should make the milk up with boiling water,' she said. 'You can't stop a woman from bottle-feeding because there might be a bug in the formula milk.'

Now this to me makes sense, and kind of chimes a little with what Ellie Lee and Joan Wolf had to say. Okay, they are unlikely to stay on the same page as the RCM for very long (even this one). And obviously Janet believed that hygiene was key while the other two thought it was less significant in developed countries. Either way Janet has worked as a midwife for over 30 years and seen a hell of a lot more babies than I have.

So, assuming one decides to accept the official advice about bottle-feeding... hang on, what exactly *is* the advice?

I told Janet Fyle about all the conflicting information that seems to vary from midwife to midwife. Shouldn't happen, she said. Information is made available to both midwives and parents. Ah yes – those leaflets again.

But do these overworked midwives in understaffed positions you're telling me about have the time to sit down with a pamphlet between contractions, especially if it's about something they don't believe in anyway?

'They *should*,' Janet said. 'We can't mix what we think women should be doing with their babies with safety information. We can't just turn our backs and say, "I don't believe you should be doing this so therefore I won't find the information."

'There are two issues midwives have – number one, don't force the woman to feed the baby the way you, the midwife, wants; number two, give her proper information. I don't think that takes a long time.'

I can't help but think that if more midwives were like Janet Fyle, I wouldn't have needed to write this book.

'How about all the women who can't breastfeed?' I asked. 'Why are they made to feel so bad?'

Janet blamed peer pressure.

'A woman might think, *she's done it; how come I can't?* I don't think this is coming from the midwife. What will hit them is pressure from other women,' she said. 'When I go to practise as a midwife – I am first a midwife – I can't see them making a woman do stuff she doesn't want to do.'

I was glad to hear her say she still practises midwifery because I was starting to wonder whether Janet was living in a parallel universe. It's one I would quite like to live in, by the sound of things. But she has not locked herself away in a comfortable office and is still an active midwife. Here. In this country.

I told her about the women in this book – Jo and her agonising mastitis, Shalene and her breast surgery. Why were they told to just keep trying?

Janet didn't put up much of an argument. 'It's okay to say, "oh, we need you to keep trying", but you can't say that when you can't see what effect it is having,' she conceded.

We reverted back again to the lack of staff, the lack of continuity, the way nobody has a single dedicated midwife that sees them through from start to finish (unless you can afford to hire a doula, which can cost anything up to £1,000).

I told Janet about another Zoe in this book, the one who cried while telling her story even though it all happened more than four years ago. Janet was worried.

'When women are genuinely upset about it, we need to talk about it and do so in a rational way,' she answered.

I can't help but feel encouraged that we might spark a conversation that desperately needs to be had, in some corner of the Royal College of Midwives and then elsewhere. Not by me, I hasten to add. I've done my bit, I think. But hopefully by someone who can actually do something other than swear like a trooper and get mad enough to start writing a book when they have a two-week-old baby and disappointingly small boobs.

When I listened back to our conversation, I felt sad. I thought war had been declared on bottle-feeders. I thought it had been started by midwives and flamed by the internet. Janet wrongfooted me by being so damned reasonable. I am also learning that as a parent everything you do is up for grabs to be judged by others. Vaccinations, sleeping arrangements, clothing, haircuts... perhaps the breastfeeding issue hurts so much because it's a brutal baptism of fire. Your first experience of being judged as either 'us' or 'them'. But I do strongly believe that a bit of bedside manner wouldn't go astray in those crucial early days.

However you feed your child, you should feel bloody proud of yourself, and you should have access to the information you need to do the job properly.

And even if you are the world's biggest control freak (I am almost certainly up there in the top ten), you should also accept that not everything is your fault.

Right at the end of our epic phone call Janet Fyle said something to me that could almost have been an alternative title to this book. It certainly silenced my inner control freak, which is no mean feat. It's so easy to forget that you may be the chef but you are not the diner in this uber-organic and very exclusive restaurant – and if your tiny little client can't or won't use the cutlery, there's not a lot you can do about it.

'It's not women who breastfeed,' she said. 'It's babies.'

Birth, Boobs and Bad Advice

THE BLOG

Want more?
There are more breastfeeding battles and discussions on the blog:

birthboobsandbadadvice.wordpress.com
See you there.....

SOURCES

Page 9
Commission Directive 2006/141/EC of 22 December 2006, based on a UNICEF/World Health Organisation treaty from 1981 called the International Code of Marketing of Breast-Milk Substitutes: http://eur-lex.europa.eu/LexUriServ/LexUriServ.do?uri=CELEX:32006L0141:EN:NOT
wonky vegetables – www.time.com/time/health/article/0,8599,1859905,00.html
2010 eggs by the dozen draft legislation – www.thegrocer.co.uk/fmcg/unit-sales-to-be-axed-by-mad-new-eu-law/210390.article
NICE website: www.nice.org.uk/nicemedia/live/10988/30146/30146.pdf

Page 10
Infant mortality figures: http://2011.census.gov.uk/files/pdf/1341-Snapshots_from_thecensus_years.pdf)
'nursery recipes': www.birdsontheblog.co.uk/what-you-should-feed-your-babies-and-toddlers-—100-years-ago/

Page 11
British Library: www.bl.uk/learning/langlit/booksforcooks/1900s/1900sfood.html
The British Association for Parenteral and Enteral Nutrition: www.bapen.org.uk/

Page 29
UK Drugs in Lactation Advisory Service: www.ukmi.nhs.uk/activities/specialistServices/default.asp?pageRef=2
British Thyroid Association: www.british-thyroid-association.org
Cardiff University School of Medicine: http://medicine.cf.ac.uk/

Page 32
Ina May's Guide to Childbirth, by Ina May Gaskin, Vermillion, ISBN 009 1924154

Page 50
Ellie Lee article: Mums who choose bottle over breastfeeding 'demonised' (17 december 2010): www.bbc.co.uk/news/health-12008913

Page 51
Ten Steps to Successful Breastfeeding: www.unicef.org.uk/BabyFriendly/Health-Professionals/Going-Baby-Friendly/Maternity/Ten-Steps-to-Successful-Breastfeeding/)
The International Code of Marketing of Breastmilk Substitutes: http://www.unicef.org.uk/BabyFriendly/Health-Professionals/Going-Baby-Friendly/Maternity/The-International-Code-of-Marketing-of-Breastmilk-Substitutes-/

Page 52
Report of women being sterilised in Uzbekistan, www.bbc.co.uk/news/magazine-17612550
Hitler Among The Germans, Rudolph Binion, published by Northern Illinois University Press (January 1, 1984) ISBN-10: 0875805310

Page 63
Neonatal Formulary information about bromocriptine : www.neonatalformulary.com/pdfs/archive/bromocriptine.pdf

Page 90
Bottled Up: How the Way We Feed Babies Has Come to Define Motherhood, and Why It Shouldn't, Suzanne Barston, University of California Press, ISBN 05 2027 0231

Page 92
CBS news report www.cbsnews.com/8301-504763_162-57347761-10391704/wal-mart-awaits-infant-formula-test-results-after-baby-dies/

Page 104
Is Breast Best? Joan B Wolf, New York University Press, ISBN 08 14794815

Page 106
Belarus study: www.health.harvard.edu/fhg/fhgupdate/R/R1.shtml

Birth, Boobs and Bad Advice

ACKNOWLEDGEMENTS

Thanks to all the ladies in this book who relived their breastfeeding sorrows again so that we could spread the word. To Ellie Lee and Joan Wolf for taking it seriously, to Janet Fyle at the RCM for responding with dignity and intelligence; to Charlie Wilson (www.thebookspecialist.com) for her thoughtful editing and for not minding the sweary bits; to my family and friends for putting up with me going on about this book at every opportunity (even those who fundamentally disagree with me).

To my sister Aimee for so much more than the text message! Thank you Helen Jackson for the blurb, Sophia Blackwell for the eagle eyes, PR superstar Polly Berrido for the wonderful press release and Gary Lonergan the fabulous graphic designer for his InDesign wizardry (www.garylonergan.com).

Finally, big kisses to my gorgeous husband Reece (www.reecedeville.com) who designed the cover and helped me every step of the way after going through it all with me when our little man was born.

Birth, Boobs and Bad Advice

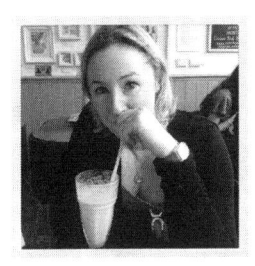

ABOUT THE AUTHOR

Zoe Kleinman is a thirty-something journalist and broadcaster. Born in London, she now lives in Hampshire with her husband and son, and recently fulfilled a lifelong ambition to feed penguins at a local zoo.